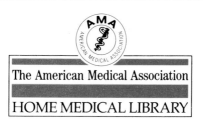

The American Medical Association

HOME MEDICAL LIBRARY

YOUR
HEART

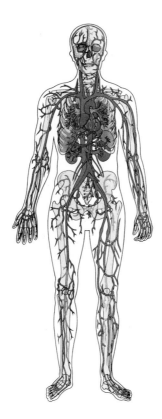

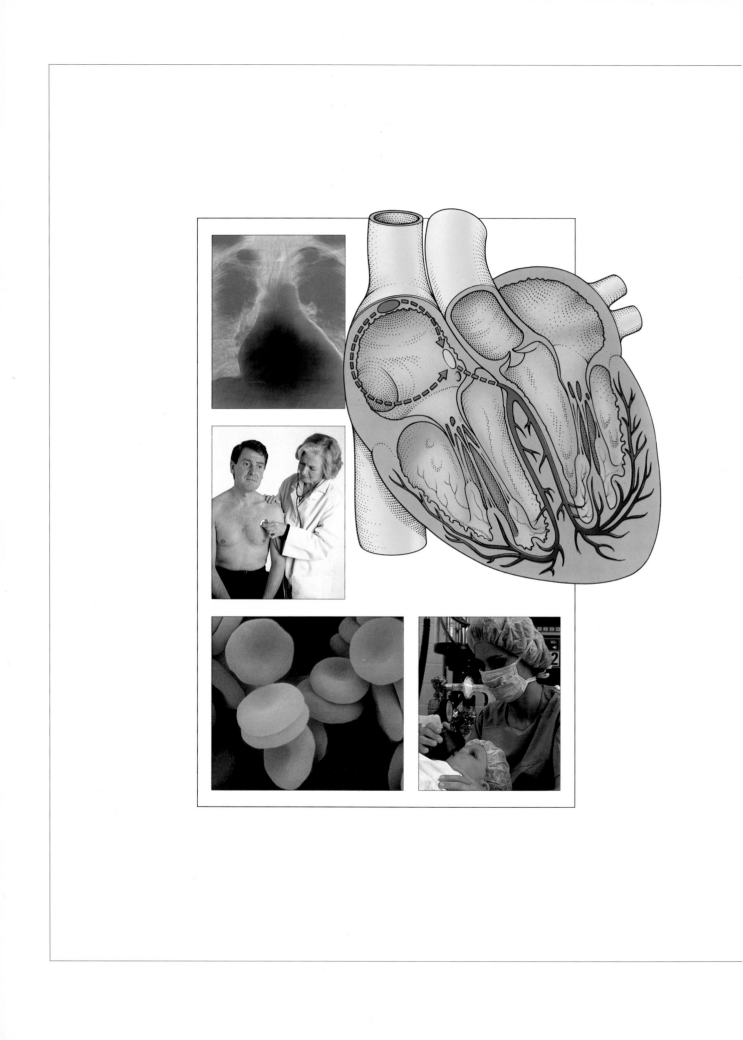

THE AMERICAN
MEDICAL ASSOCIATION

YOUR
HEART

Medical Editor
CHARLES B. CLAYMAN, MD

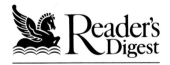

THE READER'S DIGEST ASSOCIATION, INC.
Pleasantville, New York/Montreal

The AMA Home Medical Library was created and produced
by Dorling Kindersley, Ltd., in association with the
American Medical Association.

The information in this book reflects current medical knowledge. The
recommendations and information are appropriate in most cases;
however, they are not a substitute for medical diagnosis. For specific
information concerning your personal medical condition, the AMA
suggests that you consult a physician.

The names of organizations, products, or alternative therapies appearing
in this book are given for informational purposes only. Their inclusion
does not imply AMA endorsement, nor does the omission of any
organization, product, or alternative therapy indicate AMA disapproval.

The AMA Home Medical Library is distinct from and unrelated to the
series of health books published by Random House, Inc., in conjunction
with the American Medical Association under the names "The AMA Home
Reference Library" and "The AMA Home Health Library."

Library of Congress Cataloging in Publication Data

Your heart / the American Medical Association : medical editor,
    Charles B. Clayman.
        p.   cm. — (American Medical Association home medical library)
        Includes bibliographical references.
        ISBN 0-89577-344-9
        1. Heart — Diseases — Popular works. 2. Coronary heart disease —
Prevention. I. Clayman, Charles B. II. American Medical
Association. III. Series: American Medical Association. AMA home
medical library.
        RC672.Y68 1989
        616. 1'2 — dc20   89-24074
                                                                      CIP

FOREWORD

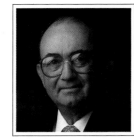

Heart disease is the leading cause of death in developed countries, a fact that has been documented for several decades. Each year coronary heart disease kills thousands of people who were otherwise in good health. Premature death from coronary heart disease can be avoided. This volume of the AMA Home Medical Library explains in detail how heart disease varies in different countries around the world and why certain changes you can make to your way of life will reduce your risk of suffering a heart attack. Later in this book, we describe how the healthy heart works to maintain the circulation of blood around the body. We also review the range of disorders that can affect this powerful muscle and its blood vessels – from birth defects and faulty heart valves to the degeneration that can affect your arteries in old age.

We are pleased to report that medical science is winning the war against heart disease. In the US, deaths from heart disease have been cut by a third since 1950. Much of this improvement is due to healthy life-style changes that include exercising regularly, managing stress, controlling weight, eating for a healthy heart, and giving up smoking. However, some improvement is due to significant advances in medical knowledge and technique. In the last 10 to 20 years an array of new diagnostic methods have been developed for assessing the health of your heart. Additional chapters in this volume describe these techniques and explain how you can benefit from them and from the exciting recent advances in treatment, including surgery to open up blocked heart arteries and the use of "clot-busting" drugs. We are not immortal, and people will continue to die of heart disease. But with the use of current medical knowledge and preventive measures many of us and our loved ones can enjoy healthy, active lives that are free of the symptoms of heart disease.

JAMES H. SAMMONS, MD
Executive Vice President, American Medical Association

CONTENTS

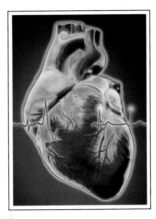

CHAPTER ONE

FIGHTING HEART DISEASE

INTRODUCTION

A WORLDWIDE
CAMPAIGN

ATHEROSCLEROSIS –
THE SILENT
EPIDEMIC

ESPITE THE CLAIMS of poets and song-writers, the heart is not the seat of the emotions. In reality, it is a tough, hard-working, muscular pump, slightly larger than a clenched fist, that is designed to circulate blood around the body by beating about 70 times a minute, 24 hours a day, for 80 years or more. It speeds up most responsively as you exert yourself, when it may be pumping five times the normal amount of blood, slows down when you are asleep, and can cope with devastating damage to its valves, muscle, and timing system. Quite an achievement. Yet, if it stops beating for even as little as 4 minutes, the result is death or irreversible major brain damage for its owner. It has long been known that the heart, though a highly resilient organ, is susceptible to disease. In the past, a common cause was rheumatic fever, which often damaged the heart valves in childhood and led to prolonged illness in later years. In the middle third of the 20th century, however, a disturbing new trend was noticed in world health statistics. Coronary heart disease, in which the heart muscle is damaged, sometimes fatally, by a blockage in the arteries that supply it, had become the number one cause of premature death in developed countries.

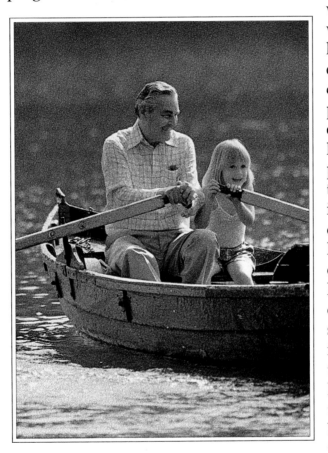

Intensive research identified coronary heart disease as largely the consequence of some key risk factors. Sedentary living, little exercise, a diet rich in saturated fats, smoking, high blood pressure, obesity, high blood cholesterol levels, diabetes, family history of heart disease, and too much tension and stress were pinpointed as contributory factors in the development of the disease. The increasingly grim statistics were a warning that we could continue to live in that fashion only at our peril. This chapter looks at the pattern of heart disease worldwide and how, in particular, people throughout the world are dealing with the number one killer, coronary heart disease. The chapter explains how the disease is caused by atherosclerosis, a narrowing of the arteries that can act like a lethal time bomb on the heart and the brain. It introduces the preventive measures that more and more people are adopting to safeguard their hearts. A greater awareness of risk factors and the sophisticated treatments that have been developed to alleviate existing heart conditions are helping us fight heart disease. It is encouraging that no country has achieved as much in this regard as the US; over the last 30 years, coronary-related deaths have been reduced by a full one third.

A WORLDWIDE CAMPAIGN

The design of the heart is virtually perfect – no man-made artificial heart has even begun to approach the performance of the natural organ. Yet the stresses, strains, and life-styles of many people in developed countries, including the US, are such that their hearts become prematurely diseased. Heart disease has become the number one killer in all social classes and all races living in North America and the northern European countries. In addition, fatalities due to heart disease are rising fast in many developing countries in Asia, Africa, and South America. Heart disease is epidemic. Because of this there is a worldwide campaign to teach people the preventive measures that promote good health and safeguard their hearts.

THE PATTERN OF HEART DISEASE

Overall, heart disease accounts for about one third of all fatalities in adult life. In 1984, for example, 766,130 people in the

WORLDWIDE DEATH RATES FROM CORONARY HEART DISEASE

The death rates from coronary heart disease in a selection of countries are given for three periods of time. From left to right they are 1960 to 1964, 1970 to 1974, and 1980 to 1984. The figures are per 100,000 of the population and are standardized to accommodate the differing age structures in different countries.

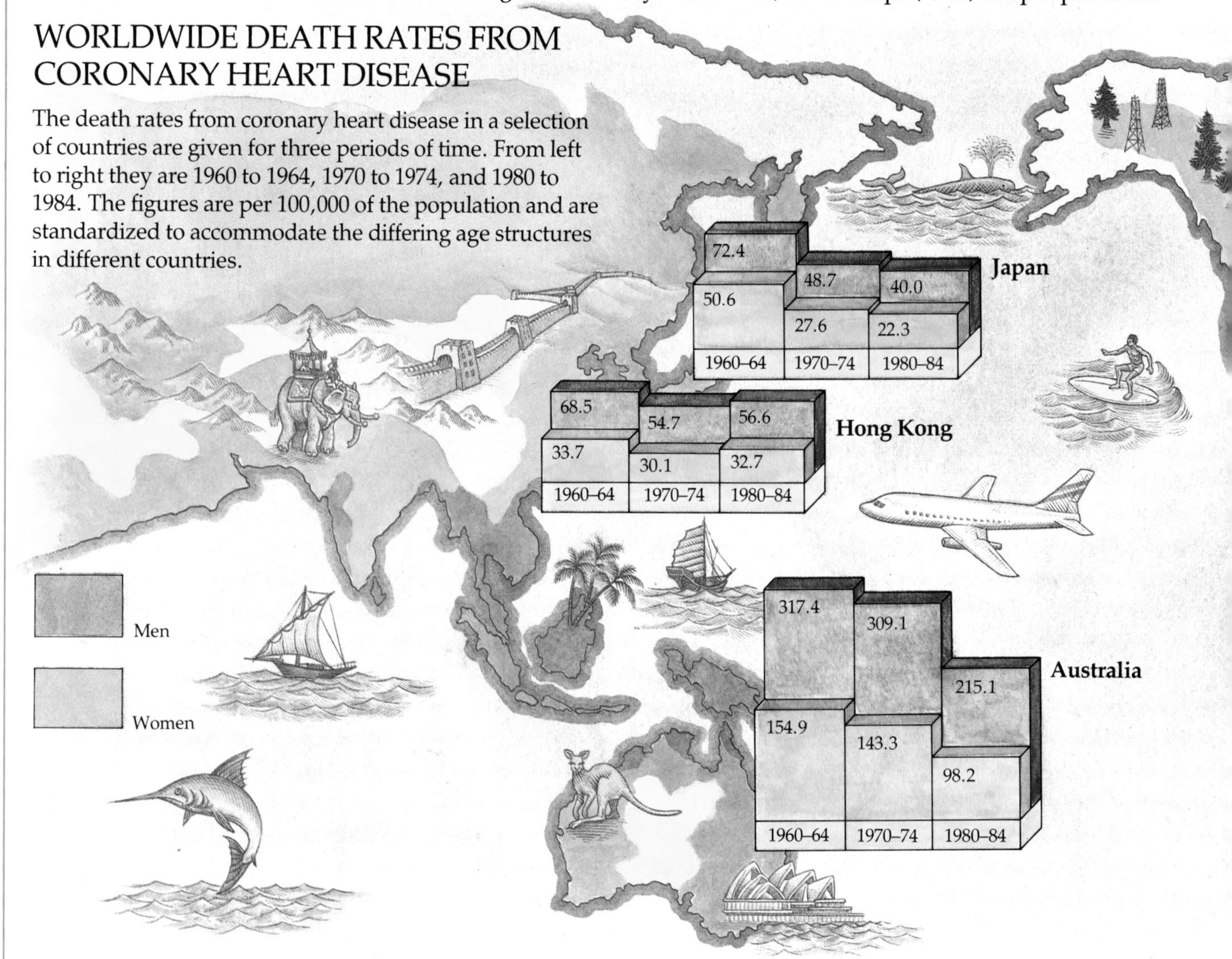

Men

Women

Japan

	1960–64	1970–74	1980–84
	72.4	48.7	40.0
	50.6	27.6	22.3

Hong Kong

	1960–64	1970–74	1980–84
	68.5	54.7	56.6
	33.7	30.1	32.7

Australia

	1960–64	1970–74	1980–84
	317.4	309.1	215.1
	154.9	143.3	98.2

US died as a result of heart disease. Many of these deaths were premature – occurring between the ages of 40 and 60, the time of life when men and women are often shouldering heavy family and work responsibilities.

Coronary heart disease

Most of the premature deaths were caused by coronary heart disease – a condition in which fatty deposits develop on the walls of the coronary arteries that supply blood to the heart muscle. The buildup of these deposits leads to narrowing (atherosclerosis) and eventually may lead to the formation of a blood clot (thrombosis) in one of the arteries. The narrowing or blood clot deprives the muscle of oxygen-rich blood and may manifest itself in several ways. Narrowing may cause angina – an oppressive tightness or dull, aching pain in the chest that comes on with exertion and is relieved by rest. A clot obstructing the channel may be the underlying cause of angina that occurs at rest or may precipitate a heart attack (sometimes called a coronary thrombosis). Coronary heart disease can also cause progressive ill health through heart failure – a gradual loss of efficiency in the heart's pumping action – or sudden death from a disturbance in the electrical system that controls the action of the heart.

National patterns of heart disease
The varying rates of death from coronary heart disease in several countries are shown in the map below. Note how the rates in the US, United Kingdom, Finland, and Australia, where high levels of saturated fats are consumed, are consistently high compared to those of Hong Kong, Japan, Costa Rica, Italy, and Uruguay. Notice also how the death rates fell in nearly all the countries between the early 1960s and the early 1980s. The reduction in the death rate in the US was particularly steep.

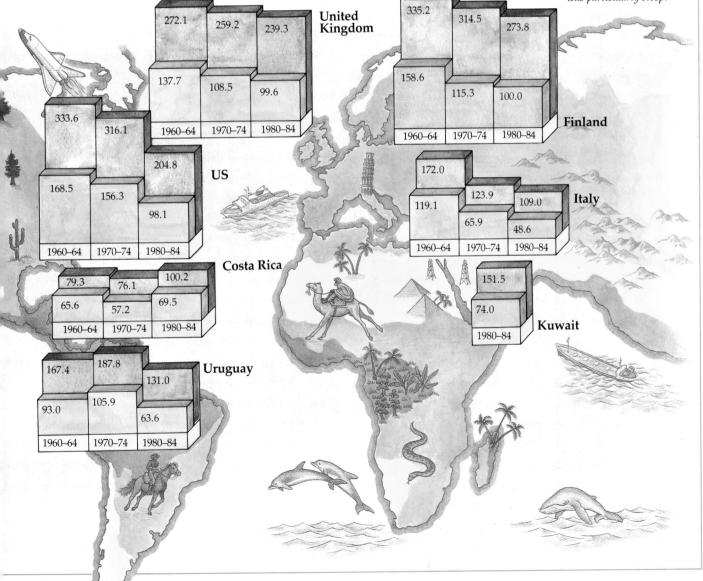

United Kingdom

	1960–64	1970–74	1980–84
	272.1	259.2	239.3
	137.7	108.5	99.6

Finland

	1960–64	1970–74	1980–84
	335.2	314.5	273.8
	158.6	115.3	100.0

US

	1960–64	1970–74	1980–84
	333.6	316.1	204.8
	168.5	156.3	98.1

Italy

	1960–64	1970–74	1980–84
	172.0	123.9	109.0
	119.1	65.9	48.6

Costa Rica

	1960–64	1970–74	1980–84
	79.3	76.1	100.2
	65.6	57.2	69.5

Kuwait

	1980–84
	151.5
	74.0

Uruguay

	1960–64	1970–74	1980–84
	167.4	187.8	131.0
	93.0	105.9	63.6

Heart problems in the young and old

Coronary heart disease is not the only cause of heart-related deaths. One child in every 100 born alive has some structural fault in the heart. Most of these defects can now be treated successfully, but congenital heart defects continue to account for many stillbirths and very early deaths. In the aged, the heart valves may deteriorate and the body's major blood vessels gradually lose their elasticity – a condition called hardening of the arteries, which leads to several life-threatening conditions.

The heart may also be affected by hormonal disorders, which can disturb its rhythm. Untreated high blood pressure can strain and enlarge the heart over a period of years. In addition, some infections, a high alcohol intake, and some vitamin deficiencies may damage the heart muscle.

Help for the heart

Medicine has made great strides in the treatment of all types of heart disease.

Reaching the people
The remarkable reduction in coronary fatalities by one third in the US was achieved partly by poster campaigning.

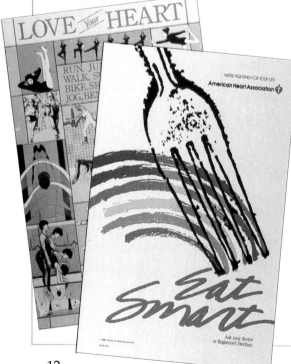

Surgical and drug treatments for coronary heart disease have literally given new life to many victims. Doctors today can repair congenital heart defects, clean out obstructed arteries, and repair or replace most narrowed or degenerated heart valves. A heart that has virtually ceased to function can now be replaced through a heart transplant operation.

PREVENTIVE MEASURES

Despite recent breakthroughs, many people will continue to die of the two main atherosclerosis-related conditions – coronary heart disease and stroke. But the age at which people die of these conditions can be extended and the quality of life in old age can be improved.

Thirty years ago, a group of scientists took a stand against the disease that was striking down their contemporaries, many of whom were in the prime of life. They outlined the "anticoronary lifestyle," a set of rules that protect the body from heart disease. Their ideas have been promoted by doctors in the US with two additions – screening tests for raised blood levels of cholesterol and regular checkups for high blood pressure.

Success measured in lives

For the past 20 years this sustained campaign of health education, and the early identification and treatment of people in high-risk categories, has gradually cut the death rate from coronary heart disease in the US by one third. In 1960, the US was near the top of the international table of death rates from coronary heart disease; today, the US is down toward the middle of that list. Most of the improvement has come from Americans taking the initiative to live a healthier lifestyle, especially by quitting smoking, maintaining a proper diet, and exercising more, and from improved medical treatment. Nevertheless, with 4,000 heart attacks occurring each day in the US, there is no excuse for complacency.

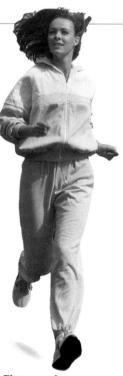

Fit to survive
Quitting smoking and lowering your blood pressure and cholesterol level in conjunction with regular aerobic exercise results in a healthy heart.

THE ANTICORONARY LIFE-STYLE

The rules to follow are:

◆ **Do not smoke.**

◆ **Follow a prudent diet, low in saturated fat and high in fiber** – this type of diet also helps you keep your weight down and contributes to a trim appearance.

◆ **Exercise regularly** – this can and should be both physically and socially enjoyable.

◆ **Manage stress and tension** –which also will reduce any anxiety and encourage a more relaxed life.

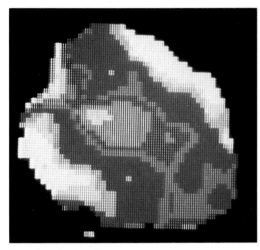

Imaging the heart
New technology provides information about the health of the heart. The red areas in the radionuclide scan above show the regions containing the most blood.

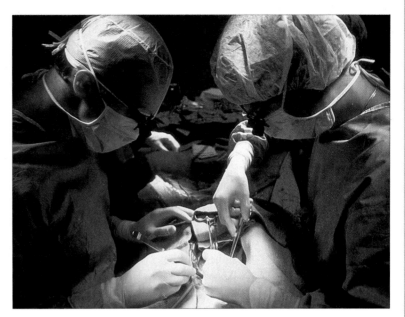

TECHNOLOGY AND THE HEART

After World War II, the wave of technological advance that brought color TV, computers, and space travel brought advances in diagnostic techniques. These included the use of monitoring devices for evaluating alterations in the heart rhythm, ultrasound for visualizing structural changes, and angiography, which permits evaluation of the blood vessels. In addition, effective drugs were produced to lower blood pressure, lower cholesterol, dissolve blood clots forming in the arteries, combat irregularities in the heartbeat, and strengthen the power of the failing heart.

Operating on the heart

Surgical treatment was transformed by the development of the heart-lung machine, which took over the task of oxygenating and circulating the blood during a heart operation. Using this apparatus, the surgeon could stop the patient's heart while he or she repaired it, making it possible to correct more congenital heart defects, replace damaged heart valves with artificial substitutes, and use a vein or artery graft to bypass blocked or narrowed sections of the coronary arteries.

New "clot-busting" (thrombolytic) drugs can dissolve blood clots and restore the flow of blood to a threatened region of the heart muscle. A narrowed coronary artery today can be stretched open again in an operation called transluminal balloon angioplasty. And heart transplantation is now a successful treatment for certain patients whose hearts are too damaged for normal life.

Heart transplants
First successfully completed by Dr. Christiaan Barnard in 1967, the heart transplant operation requires a heart-lung machine to supply oxygenated blood to the body while the patient's heart is removed and a new one is inserted. More than 80 percent of patients survive beyond a year after the operation.

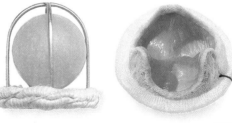

Replacing nature's failing parts
A malfunctioning heart valve can be replaced surgically with a substitute made of plastic and metal (above) or taken from a pig or cadaver (above right). Patients with certain disorders of the heart's electrical control system can be restored to health by an electronic pacemaker (right) or an automatic defibrillator.

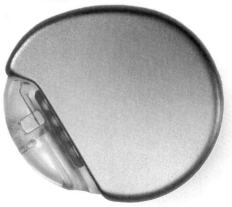

ATHEROSCLEROSIS – THE SILENT EPIDEMIC

Advances in surgical treatments, patient monitoring in intensive-care units, and the drugs used to fight heart disease have cut the death rate in heart attack patients admitted to hospitals. However, almost half of all deaths from coronary heart disease and more than half of all strokes occur suddenly, without warning, in people who had no previous symptoms. These are the victims of the "silent" epidemic of the 20th century – atherosclerosis.

NARROWING OF THE ARTERIES

A dictionary definition of atherosclerosis might be "a disease of the arterial wall in which the inner layer thickens, causing narrowing of the channel and thus impairing blood flow." In practice, atherosclerosis is a disease of human behavior. It affects people who eat more than they need, people who smoke cigarettes, and people whose lives rarely require any prolonged physical exertion. Such a life-style encourages the accumulation in the blood of fats and the oily substance cholesterol. The mixture of fats and cholesterol infiltrates the lining of the arteries, narrowing and damaging them, so that under the microscope they look like hot-water pipes clogged by mineral deposits. Once narrowed, the arteries are vulnerable to total blockage by a blood clot.

Narrowing of the arteries does not affect the body's blood vessels equally; the pattern varies from one person to another. Most commonly, the narrowing takes place in the coronary arteries that supply blood to the heart, resulting in coronary heart disease. However, in some people, the coronary arteries remain fairly healthy while there is a severe narrowing of the arteries that supply blood to the brain (a major cause of stroke). In others, the narrowing may be severe in the arteries that supply blood to the legs. This can cause pain in the legs while walking and gangrene in the feet. If an artery to a kidney is narrowed, a rise in blood pressure can result.

Who gets atherosclerosis?

The pathologists who examined bodies after death and built the foundation of medical science in the 19th century paid little attention to atherosclerosis, although they did describe it in their reports. Most of the bodies they examined were of people who had died young or in middle age. Survival past the age of 60 was far from usual until this century.

When the number of deaths from coronary heart disease and stroke began to show an increase in the late 1930s and the 1940s, medical scientists had little understanding of the underlying cause of this change in pattern. One of the first clues was discovered when they re-

Atheroma
The fatty material known as atheroma, shown below in the lining of an arterial wall, consists mainly of cholesterol, blood lipids (fats), and fatty acid compounds known as triglycerides. Science has not established indisputably that a low cholesterol intake in the diet can help prevent atherosclerosis, but all the evidence suggests that it does.

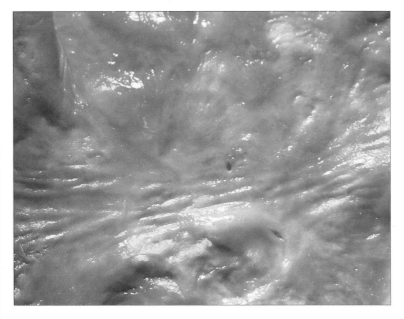

HOW DOES ATHEROSCLEROSIS OCCUR?

In all people, atheroma (a fatty deposit containing cholesterol) builds up to one degree or another under the lining of the arteries from childhood onward. Lipoproteins, which carry the atheroma-forming cholesterol, penetrate the lining of the arteries and become trapped behind the lining, causing inflammation and scarring. Large patches, known as atheromatous plaques, then build up over the damaged areas. Blood clots can form on the atheromatous plaque if the surface of the plaque becomes irregular or if the flow of blood becomes sluggish. In addition, calcium can harden the plaques, a condition described by the term "hardening of the arteries." Over the years, the plaques grow larger, until gradually the artery narrows or is blocked completely, clogged by the accumulated material.

Superior vena cava

Aorta

Left main coronary artery

Pulmonary artery

Left circumflex artery

Right coronary artery

Left anterior descending artery

Supplying the heart

Two main coronary arteries stem from the aorta to supply the oxygen- and nutrient-rich blood that feeds the heart. The larger, left coronary artery has two branches (the left circumflex artery and the left anterior descending artery), which supply blood to the front and left sides of the heart. The right coronary artery circles around the right side to the back. A network of tributaries branches off the arteries to penetrate deep into the heart muscle. A blockage in any part of the system can cause death of part of the heart muscle – better known as a heart attack. Its severity depends on how much of the heart is deprived of blood.

Developing atheromatous plaque

Damaged arterial wall

Danger sites
Atheromatous plaques often occur at arterial branches (bifurcations), the point at which dividing streams of blood create natural turbulence. The rough, damaged surfaces of the growing plaques further increase the turbulence. The clotting mechanism of the blood is triggered by this agitation, and the scene is set for the formation of a potentially lethal blood clot (thrombus). Unless the clot is dissolved, it can enlarge and block the artery, depriving the organ it supplies of oxygenated blood.

Fibrous cap

Fatty core

A growing plaque
An established plaque grows through a buildup of platelets (particles in the blood that assist in blood coagulation) and white blood cells. A part of the plaque may rupture, leading to clot formation on the surface of the plaque and resulting in blockage of the vessel (coronary artery occlusion) and heart attack.

viewed the data on the death rates among different countries. The scientists observed that coronary heart disease is very common in some technically advanced countries – notably the United Kingdom, Finland, and the US – but it is far less common in other comparably advanced countries such as Italy and Japan. However, when Italian or Japanese people came to live in the US, within a generation their descendants had rates of coronary heart disease as high as those of their fellow Americans. This suggested that environment and life-style were more significant than nationality in determining a person's susceptibility to heart disease. This was further confirmed when autopsies performed on American soldiers who had died in the Korean and Vietnam wars revealed varying stages of atherosclerosis.

THE LIFE-STYLE LINK

Diet is one of the primary life-style factors identified as a cause of heart disease. However, while some people living in developed countries and eating certain foods suffer severe atherosclerosis, others living in the same country and eating a similar range of foods do not. Diet is clearly important, especially its fat and cholesterol content, but recent research has identified other risk factors.

It is known that heart disease due to atherosclerosis often runs in families. If a man has a heart attack while in his 40s, his brothers and cousins are at increased risk of suffering a heart attack too. In these families, a biochemical variation in the way the body processes fats leads to very high levels of cholesterol in the

DIETARY FATS AND OILS – WHICH ONES ARE SAFE?

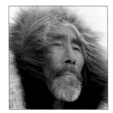

Eskimos consume more fats in their diet than any other people in the world, yet heart disease develops in very few individuals. The explanation for this apparent paradox is that the fats, which mostly come from seal blubber or fish, are unsaturated and of a type known as the omega-3 fatty acids, which seem to be linked to a low incidence of heart disease among Eskimos. All unsaturated fats are liquid or semi-liquid at room temperature (right). In countries with low rates of heart disease, the people have lower cholesterol levels and either eat relatively little animal fat (as in Japan and other Asian countries) or eat mostly unsaturated fat. Also, fish rather than meat is often preferred.

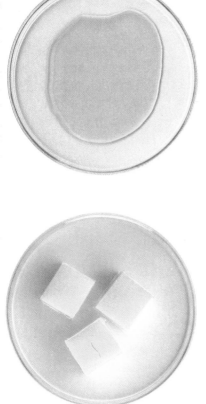

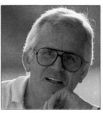

Americans and people living in northern European countries often have high levels of cholesterol in their blood, which accounts in part for their high rates of coronary heart disease. Like the Eskimos, they eat a considerable amount of fat, but the fats are saturated. These fats are solid at room temperature (right) and contribute to the formation by the liver of unhealthy cholesterol, which ultimately makes its way into the walls of the arteries. Saturated fats are found in animal sources, tropical oils such as palm and coconut oils, and dairy products. Saturated fats encourage the formation of atheroma, the substance that builds up in the arteries and leads to heart and arterial disease.

blood – a condition known as familial hypercholesterolemia. Other inherited biochemical disorders in which the blood contains too much fat lead similarly to early death from heart attack.

Recent advances in understanding the role of heredity have led to treatment to reduce the dangerously high cholesterol levels in susceptible people. However, in most cases, these disorders have few symptoms; for treatment to be given in time the disorders must first be recognized. Everyone should have a cholesterol test at age 20. People who have a blood relative in whom heart disease developed before age 50 should notify their doctor at the time of the test.

The gender factor

Another factor to take into account is gender. Deaths from coronary heart disease before age 60 are much more common in men than in women; between the ages of 45 and 50, men are four times more likely to die of it than women. The explanation for this imbalance seems to be that female sex hormones have a protective effect. After the menopause, women become much more susceptible to coronary heart disease; by age 70, the sex difference has disappeared.

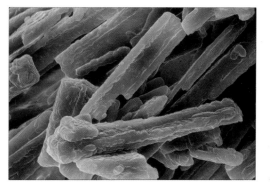

Reducing the risk

If a sample group of several thousand young men were examined by doctors, some would show signs of early coronary heart disease. Research performed for 20 years or more in Europe and the US shows that deaths from coronary heart disease are more common in men who smoke cigarettes. The risk increases with the number smoked each day, and decreases when the smoker quits. The same studies show that men who weigh more than 20 percent above their recommended weight are at increased risk, as are those who have raised blood pressure. The message is that quitting smoking, staying trim, and controlling blood cholesterol and blood pressure are vital if you want to prevent or postpone atherosclerosis.

Cholesterol
The picture at left shows some waxy cholesterol crystals. The main component of atheroma, cholesterol is a fatlike substance found in most tissues. It is essential for producing new cells and certain hormones. Most of the body's cholesterol is synthesized in the liver from dietary nutrients. The body does not actually need the extra cholesterol absorbed from the meat, eggs, and dairy products we eat.

IS YOUR BLOOD CHOLESTEROL LEVEL TOO HIGH?

If the cholesterol level in your blood has not been checked in the last 5 years, ask your doctor whether you should have it measured. An abnormally high level may be a warning that you are more at risk of coronary heart disease than others in your age group. If this is the case, your doctor will probably want to check your high-density lipoprotein (HDL) cholesterol level and do a calculation of your low-density lipoprotein (LDL) cholesterol level. Although a high total level of cholesterol in

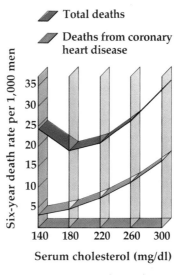

■ Total deaths

■ Deaths from coronary heart disease

Six-year death rate per 1,000 men

35
30
25
20
15
10
5

140 180 220 260 300

Serum cholesterol (mg/dl)

the blood is associated with an increased mortality from coronary heart disease (see graph at left), ongoing refinements in measuring cholesterol indicate how complex our metabolism is by showing that there are different types of cholesterol, both good and bad. LDL is the unhealthy cholesterol that infiltrates the walls of arteries to form atheroma. HDL is the healthy cholesterol, which is thought to help carry away some of the LDL cholesterol from the walls of the arteries.

CHAPTER TWO

THE ANTICORONARY LIFE-STYLE

A LOT OF HEART ATTACKS need never occur. Medical research has pinpointed several simple preventive measures that, if followed by everyone, would dramatically cut the rates of illness and death from coronary heart disease. The risk factors for coronary heart disease fall into two groups. There are those about which you can do little or nothing, like your age, sex, any history of diabetes mellitus, and any inherited tendency to heart trouble. Then there are those about which you can do a great deal. These include your diet, your weight, the amount you exercise, your blood pressure, and (possibly) the level of stress in your life and how well you are able to cope with it. Probably the most important risk factor of all is whether or not you smoke. The facts regarding most of these risk factors are irrefutable. Differing incidences of heart disease in countries with differing diets is just one of many pieces of evidence that what you eat does affect your heart. Smokers are much more likely to die of heart disease than nonsmokers. Similarly, people who exercise very little or not at all are at higher risk than the physically active. Exercise makes the heart muscle stronger, causes it to work more efficiently with less effort, helps you con-

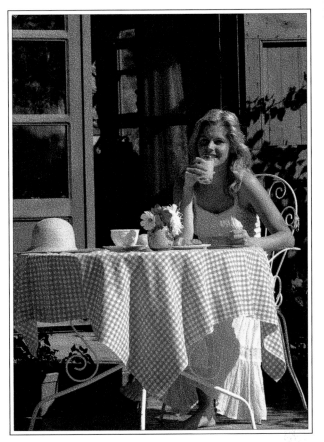

trol your weight and your blood pressure, and helps reduce levels of low-density lipoprotein (LDL) – the unhealthy cholesterol – in your blood. It also elevates blood levels of high-density lipoprotein (HDL) – the healthy cholesterol – and generally makes you feel better. The role of stress in heart disease is less direct and clear-cut, but learning how to cope successfully with a high stress level may have many unmeasured benefits in preventing heart disease.

The trend today is for people to take a much greater responsibility for their health than they used to and to rely far less on medicine as a cure-all once things have gone wrong. Prevention is, most people are now convinced, better than cure. This chapter will show you ways in which making relatively simple changes in your life-style – eating better, giving up smoking, exercising more, and coping with the unavoidable stresses in your life – can decrease your risk of heart disease. The risk factor assessment chart at the beginning of this chapter will give you an idea of how seriously you need to consider making life-style changes. The changes outlined here are easy to follow and should do much to improve not only your life expectancy but, perhaps more importantly, your quality of life.

IS YOUR HEART AT RISK?

No one can predict with absolute certainty whether heart disease will develop in later life. What is known is that heart disease is more likely to strike when certain factors are present than when they are not. To find out how much you are at risk, answer the questions below and calculate your score. It could help pinpoint changes that need to be made in the areas over which you have control.

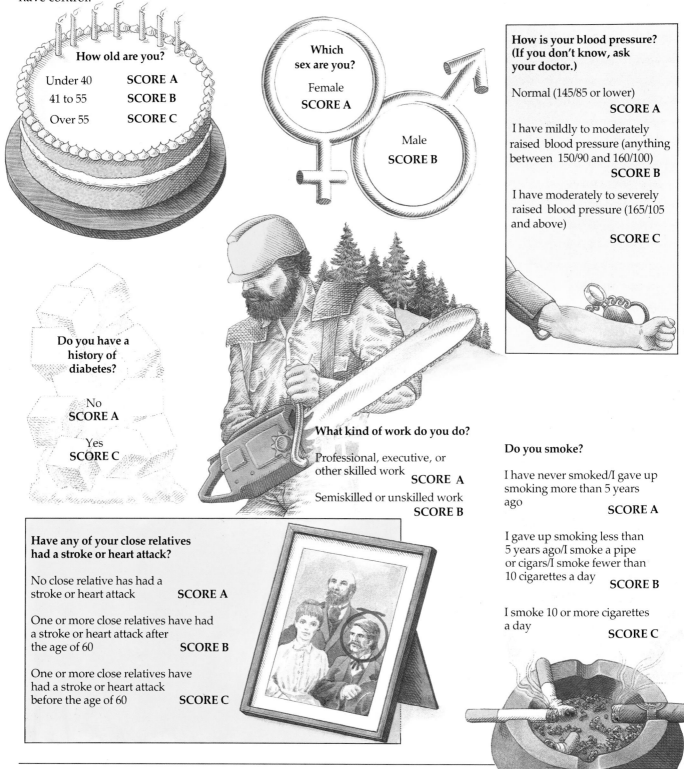

How old are you?

Under 40	**SCORE A**
41 to 55	**SCORE B**
Over 55	**SCORE C**

Which sex are you?

Female
SCORE A

Male
SCORE B

How is your blood pressure? (If you don't know, ask your doctor.)

Normal (145/85 or lower)
SCORE A

I have mildly to moderately raised blood pressure (anything between 150/90 and 160/100)
SCORE B

I have moderately to severely raised blood pressure (165/105 and above)
SCORE C

Do you have a history of diabetes?

No
SCORE A

Yes
SCORE C

What kind of work do you do?

Professional, executive, or other skilled work
SCORE A

Semiskilled or unskilled work
SCORE B

Do you smoke?

I have never smoked/I gave up smoking more than 5 years ago
SCORE A

I gave up smoking less than 5 years ago/I smoke a pipe or cigars/I smoke fewer than 10 cigarettes a day
SCORE B

I smoke 10 or more cigarettes a day
SCORE C

Have any of your close relatives had a stroke or heart attack?

No close relative has had a stroke or heart attack
SCORE A

One or more close relatives have had a stroke or heart attack after the age of 60
SCORE B

One or more close relatives have had a stroke or heart attack before the age of 60
SCORE C

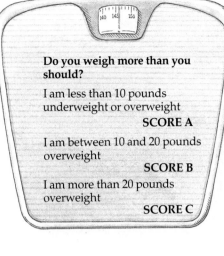

Do you weigh more than you should?

I am less than 10 pounds underweight or overweight
SCORE A

I am between 10 and 20 pounds overweight
SCORE B

I am more than 20 pounds overweight
SCORE C

Which of the following diets is closest to your own food intake?

Fish, poultry, vegetables, and fruit; infrequent red meat, cheese, cream, and butter; four or fewer eggs a week; otherwise, low-fat dairy products and polyunsaturated oils
SCORE A

Red meat three times or less a week; four to six eggs a week; fish, poultry; cheese or cream two to three times a week; daily consumption of whole milk and butter
SCORE B

One or more servings daily of red meat; seven eggs or more a week; daily consumption of butter and cheese; ½ to 1 pint of whole milk daily; more than ¼ pint of cream a week
SCORE C

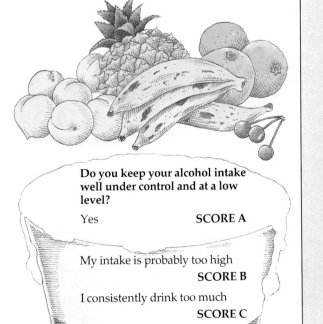

Do you keep your alcohol intake well under control and at a low level?

Yes
SCORE A

My intake is probably too high
SCORE B

I consistently drink too much
SCORE C

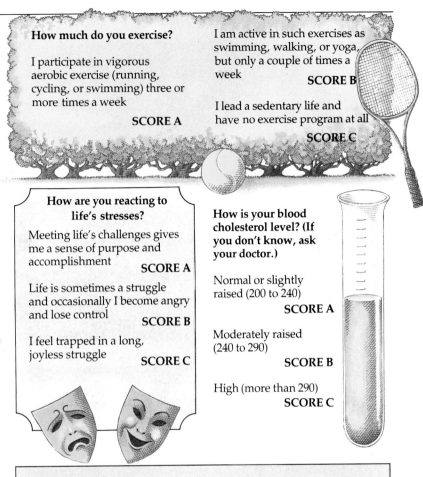

How much do you exercise?

I participate in vigorous aerobic exercise (running, cycling, or swimming) three or more times a week
SCORE A

I am active in such exercises as swimming, walking, or yoga, but only a couple of times a week
SCORE B

I lead a sedentary life and have no exercise program at all
SCORE C

How are you reacting to life's stresses?

Meeting life's challenges gives me a sense of purpose and accomplishment
SCORE A

Life is sometimes a struggle and occasionally I become angry and lose control
SCORE B

I feel trapped in a long, joyless struggle
SCORE C

How is your blood cholesterol level? (If you don't know, ask your doctor.)

Normal or slightly raised (200 to 240)
SCORE A

Moderately raised (240 to 290)
SCORE B

High (more than 290)
SCORE C

HOW DID YOU SCORE?

All As:
You are at a very low risk of heart disease, and the life-style you have chosen will continue to minimize the risk.

One to four Bs and no Cs:
There is a slight risk of heart disease. Can you eliminate one or more Bs from your score to remove that risk?

Five to seven Bs and no Cs, or up to seven Bs and one to two Cs:
There is a moderate risk that heart disease may develop. You should consider seriously whether changes could be made in your life-style to safeguard your heart and your general health. If you smoke, quit *now*.

Eight to nine Bs and/or three to four Cs:
Your score indicates that there is a high risk of heart disease now or in the future. It would be highly useful to make an appointment with your doctor to discuss how you can reduce the risk effectively. If you smoke, quit *now*.

Ten to 12 Bs or five or more Cs:
It is imperative that you ask your doctor about what can be done to help you avoid heart disease, as there is a very high risk. If you smoke, quit *now*.

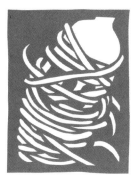

EATING FOR A HEALTHY HEART

FOLLOWING THE WRONG DIET increases your risk of heart disease. On the other hand, following the right diet can actually protect your heart and circulation. If you think that a diet that is good for your heart is dull, tasteless, and monotonous, think again. Foods that contribute to the health of your heart can be as appetizing and as fun to eat as their high-fat, low-fiber counterparts.

One of the main reasons Americans have a higher rate of coronary heart disease than, for instance, the Japanese, is that we eat too much of the wrong foods.

EAT LESS FAT

The consumption of fat in developed countries like the US is very high, and it is believed that most sedentary people would benefit by cutting that consumption by a quarter to a half. But the problem is not as simple as that; it is complicated by the fact that there is more than one kind of fat.

What kind of fat?

There are three main categories of fat in the diet – saturated, monounsaturated, and polyunsaturated. Saturated fats, which include butter, lard, the fat of meats, and palm and coconut oils, tend to raise the level of cholesterol in the blood. Cholesterol is essential for the normal functioning of the body, but high levels of low-density lipoprotein (LDL) – the unhealthy cholesterol – accelerate the build-up of deposits of atheroma on arterial walls, which, in turn, leads to heart disease.

Cholesterol
Even a moderately increased level of low-density lipoprotein (LDL) cholesterol in the blood for long periods of time can increase your risk of heart disease. Cholesterol is absorbed directly from certain foods such as eggs, while the saturated fats in foods such as french fries are converted within the body into cholesterol. Both push up the blood's cholesterol level. If you are at risk of heart disease and wish to minimize your risk, dishes prepared as shown below are best minimized or avoided.

TWO TYPES OF FAT

Saturated fats are generally those that are solid at normal room temperature – lard, butter, and the fat found in and on meat. They tend to push up your cholesterol level most easily, with deleterious effects on the heart.

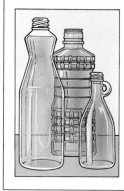

Unsaturated fats are generally those that are liquid or semiliquid at room temperature – vegetable oils (except palm and coconut oils), fish oils, and liquid margarine. They may exert a protective effect on your heart.

Unsaturated fats are found in fish and vegetable oils. These oils can be monounsaturated or polyunsaturated. Monounsaturated fats, including olive and canola oil, tend to have no effect on cholesterol. Polyunsaturated fats, including corn, sunflower, soybean, peanut, safflower, and fish oils, aid in lowering the level of cholesterol in the blood. The effect of polyunsaturated fats on blood clotting may actually play a protective role in helping to keep the walls of your arteries clear.

More than half the fat most of us eat is saturated. Cutting down on all fats is an important part of keeping your weight in line. But it is equally important that the fat you do eat is, for the most part, polyunsaturated. It may help stop the progression of existing atherosclerosis and thus help protect your heart.

High-risk groups

Certain people are at particular risk of having too much fat in their diet because they have inherited one of a group of metabolic disorders called the hyperlipidemias. These disorders cause an abnormally high level of unhealthy fats, such as very low-density lipoproteins (VLDLs) and low-density lipoproteins (LDLs), in the blood from an early age. People who have one of these disorders require a low-fat diet and sometimes drugs to lower the fat levels in their blood. The symptoms of hyperlipidemia are not always obvious. Any person with a relative who suffered a heart attack or stroke before age 50 should have a blood test in his or her early 20s to check for the presence of these disorders.

LESS SUGAR, MORE FIBER

Sugar is thought by some researchers to contribute to the risk of coronary heart disease, though the reasons for this are not clear. What is abundantly clear is that a high sugar intake plays a large part in obesity, which contributes to high blood pressure – one of the main risk factors for coronary heart disease.

Cutting down on sugar

Watch for hidden sugar in processed foods, where it may be listed under a variety of names including sucrose, dextrose, syrup, molasses, or caramel. Drink unsweetened fruit juices and dilute them with water. Eat fruit rather than a rich dessert or candy at the end of a meal or as a snack. Reduce the amount of sugar you use in recipes.

HOW TO CUT DOWN ON FAT

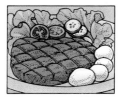

♦ Eat more grilled, baked, broiled, or boiled foods. Choose from the widest possible selection of foods, including vegetables, meat, fish, and starches.

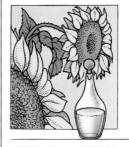

♦ Choose vegetable oils that are known to be high in polyunsaturated fats such as soybean, corn, peanut, safflower, and sunflower oils, or monounsaturated oils such as olive or canola oil. Give preference to a soft margarine that is stated to be high in polyunsaturated fats.

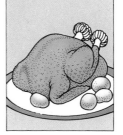

♦ Eat poultry, such as chicken and turkey, but always remove the skin and any visible fat. Select lean cuts of meat and trim all visible fat. Cook stews, soups, and casseroles slowly, skimming off the fat periodically. Allow them to cool and remove all fat before eating.

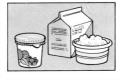

♦ Use low-fat (1 or 2 percent) or skimmed milk, low-fat yogurt, and lower-fat cheeses, such as dry cottage cheese, farmer's cheese, or a low-fat cheddar.

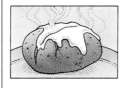

♦ Remember that much of the fat in the foods you eat is found in the sauces, gravies, and dressings. When you eat a baked potato, opt for yogurt or cottage cheese instead of sour cream.

Eat more fish
Fish with white meat, such as cod and sole, contain little fat; fatty fish, such as salmon, mackerel, and tuna, are a particularly good source of polyunsaturated oils, which are believed to have a protective effect on the circulation. It is probably beneficial to eat at least 8 ounces of fish, including fatty fish, every week.

Benefits of fiber

Fiber (what we used to call roughage) consists of the indigestible matter in the seeds, roots, shoots, leaves, flowers, and fruits of plants. The fiber in food of plant origin gives bulk to the stools and pre- vents constipation and intestinal dis- orders. As it passes through the bowel, indigestible fiber absorbs water and thereby softens the stools. It also helps control levels of cholesterol and sugar in the blood by binding with these nu- trients and partially interfering with their absorption. High-fiber foods tend to be filling without being fattening; they are particularly useful if you are trying to lose weight.

If you decide to increase your fiber intake, introduce fiber-rich foods grad- ually. A sudden change from a low- fiber diet to a high-fiber one can cause abdominal distress and flatulence.

Good sources of fiber include whole- grain cereals, whole-wheat bread, bran, pasta, brown rice, vegetables, fruits, and dried beans, peas, and lentils.

CONTROL YOUR WEIGHT

The more overweight you are, the more likely you are to get high blood pressure or diabetes, both of which can accelerate the process of atherosclerosis and increase the risk of angina and heart attacks. If you are more than 20 percent over your ideal weight, you are eating too much and exercising too little. In addition, you probably are eating the wrong foods.

One of the secondary benefits of a low- fat, low-sugar, high-fiber diet is that you are less likely to get – or to stay – fat. Spread your meals throughout the day and, in general, eat several small meals rather than one large one.

SEVEN-POINT PLAN FOR WEIGHT REDUCTION

If you are overweight, follow this seven- point plan to a trimmer appearance.

1 Eat three moderate-sized meals rather than one large meal a day.

2 Keep to reasonable helpings of poultry, fish, and lean meat.

3 Eat plenty of vegetables and salads, and finish your meals with fruit rather than rich desserts, such as pies and cakes, that have a high calorie content.

4 Eat whole-grain bread, pasta, and brown rice, but cut down on butter, oil, and margarine.

5 Avoid sugar and foods with a high sugar content.

6 Drink plenty of fluids, including water, fruit juices (preferably diluted), and tea or coffee (either black or with low-fat milk).

7 Exercise regularly, at least three times a week.

CUTTING DOWN ON SUGAR AND CALORIES

Many mass-produced foods have sugar added to them for palatability; some examples are shown below. In some cases, the sugar provides many or all of the calories in the food. Cutting down on sugar-containing foods helps prevent obesity – a risk factor for heart disease. Staying trim also helps protect against both heart disease and maturity-onset diabetes.

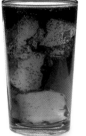

Large cola, 10 to 12 oz
Added sugar 50 g
Calories from sugar 200
Total calories 200

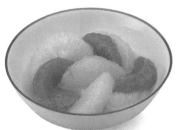

Canned grapefruit with syrup, 4 oz
Added sugar 12 g
Calories from sugar 50
Total calories 60

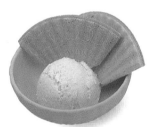

Ice-cream, one scoop
Added sugar 12 g
Calories from sugar 50
Total calories 90

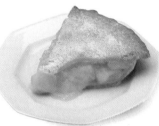

Apple pie, one slice
Added sugar 15 g
Calories from sugar 60
Total calories 350

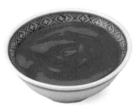

Ketchup, 1 tablespoon
Added sugar 3 g
Calories from sugar 12
Total calories 15

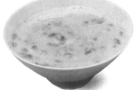

Fruit yogurt, one carton
Added sugar 17 g
Calories from sugar 70
Total calories 130

Hot dog Added sugar 9 g
Calories from sugar 35 Total calories 160

ASK YOUR DOCTOR

DIET AND YOUR HEART

Q I've changed from eating butter to polyunsaturated margarine. Is it any less fattening?

A No. Margarine is just as fattening as butter. The change may benefit your heart, but, if you are concerned about your weight, you must use all fats in moderation.

Q My son is particularly fond of hamburgers, but I've heard that they are high in fat and therefore not very good for him. Is there any way around this problem?

A It is best to buy lean ground beef or buy lean stewing beef, cut off all visible fat, and grind it yourself. Fry it without adding fat and drain off any excess fat before serving. Grilling is even better than frying.

Q I've been told I should eat less salt, because it contributes to heart disease. Is this true?

A Probably. Some experts are convinced that a high intake of salt contributes to high blood pressure in salt-sensitive people, which in turn contributes to heart disease. People with heart failure should avoid salt because sodium retains water, which aggravates the condition.

Q Are there any signs or symptoms of a higher-than-normal cholesterol level in the blood?

A Sometimes yellow fatty deposits appear on the skin, often around the eyes or over the tendons. These deposits are called xanthomas. Generally, a blood test is necessary to verify a high blood cholesterol level.

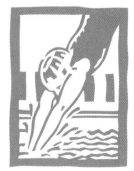

EXERCISE AND YOUR HEART

EXERCISING REGULARLY is known to reduce the risk of heart disease. It makes the heart muscle both stronger and thicker, which enables it to pump the same volume of blood around the body with fewer beats. This explains why many athletes have a remarkably slow heart rate. All evidence shows that people who exercise regularly and vigorously have a much lower chance of having a heart attack and, if they do have one, they are more likely to survive it.

Exercise increases the speed and strength of your heartbeat. At rest, your heart pumps between 10 and 12 pints of blood around your body in a minute. During exercise this rate can increase to between 18 and 70 pints per minute. If you are in shape, your heart will recover more quickly after exercise, so that your pulse returns to normal sooner.

HOW EXERCISE IMPROVES FITNESS

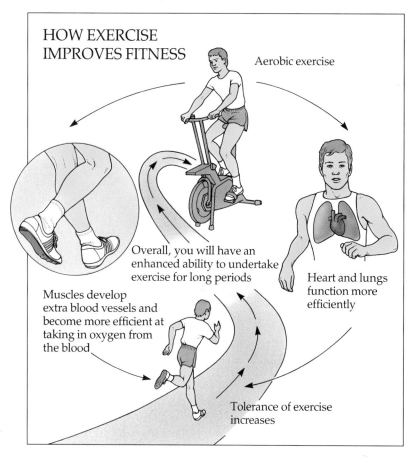

Aerobic exercise

Overall, you will have an enhanced ability to undertake exercise for long periods

Muscles develop extra blood vessels and become more efficient at taking in oxygen from the blood

Heart and lungs function more efficiently

Tolerance of exercise increases

SAFEGUARDING YOUR HEART

Regular exercise reduces the amount of unhealthy cholesterol in your bloodstream. This means that you have a lower risk of angina or of a heart attack. Another reason exercise is good for your heart is that, in conjunction with eating a healthy diet (see page 22), it helps control your weight. Exercise burns up extra calories, allows a much wider food selection, uses up fat from your body's reserves, and increases the level at which energy is burned in your tissues at rest, which helps you use excess calories when you are not exercising. People who are more than 20 percent overweight are more susceptible to high blood pressure and thus much more likely to have heart disease develop.

Exercise after a heart attack

Exercising regularly after a heart attack has been claimed by some experts to reduce your risk of having another one. Today most doctors allow you to start daily activities (such as walking short distances in your room) within a few days of a heart attack, provided you do not have any complications such as heart failure or an irregular heartbeat. Exercise levels are then gradually increased. Once the damaged area of heart muscle

HOW EXERCISE STRENGTHENS YOUR HEART

During strenuous exercise the volume of blood flowing into the heart increases. The greater volume of blood stretches the muscle, and the muscle fibers respond with a stronger, more powerful, contraction. The heart's muscle bulk increases and its blood vessels proliferate, improving the muscle's blood supply. In time, the heart becomes more efficient and pumps a greater volume of blood with each stroke, allowing the heart rate to slow down.

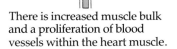

HEART OF PERSON WITH
SEDENTARY LIFE-STYLE

HEART OF PERSON WITH
ACTIVE LIFE-STYLE

Low volume of
blood from veins

Greater volume of
blood from veins

The heart muscle bulk and the blood vessel network adequately cope with the usually low pressure of blood.

There is increased muscle bulk and a proliferation of blood vessels within the heart muscle.

IS EXERCISE SAFE WITH ANGINA?

If you have angina, talk to your doctor before you begin an exercise program. Gentle exercise is recommended for most angina sufferers, many of whom are able to take regular, brisk walks. Stop exercising if any symptoms appear and never exercise if you have chest pain or severe breathlessness. Do not exercise in very cold or very hot weather or right after a heavy meal; these factors can place extra strain on your heart. Strenuous exercise, such as digging in the garden or shoveling snow, should be avoided.

has healed, which usually takes about 6 weeks, most people are allowed to return to their normal activities.

A steady pace

Start exercising with a program of slow walking, increasing your pace and the distance you walk gradually over a couple of weeks. Stop if you notice chest pain, breathlessness, palpitations, dizziness, or any other alarming symptoms. Do not exercise in very cold or very hot weather or right after a meal.

After a heart attack, many people want to know when it is safe to have sex again. Once you can climb up and down stairs without any difficulty, you should be able to cope with the exertion of sexual intercourse, although, at first, you may not be as athletic as you might have been. Bear in mind, however, that the added tensions of having sex with someone other than your regular partner may put more of a strain on your heart by causing your heart rate and blood pressure to increase dangerously.

ASK YOUR DOCTOR
EXERCISE AND THE HEALTHY HEART

Q **My wife has read that you can die suddenly during strenuous exercise. I have been training hard for a marathon and she is worried. How can I tell if I am overdoing it?**

A It is true that people die more often during exercise than when resting in bed. However, in general, people who exercise regularly live longer than those who do not. If you are concerned about your training, ask your doctor to give you a checkup. Warning signs during exercise are chest pain, pain in your neck or arms, severe breathlessness, dizziness, palpitations, or faintness.

Q **If exercise makes blood pressure go up, why does my doctor tell me to exercise to keep my blood pressure down?**

A Your blood pressure goes up during exercise because your heart is beating more forcefully. When you stop, it returns to lower than your usual blood pressure or back to normal. Regular exercise can help prevent persistently high blood pressure. It also lowers the level of cholesterol in your blood.

Q **My father died of a heart attack at age 40. Should I be worried now that I am approaching 40?**

A Anyone over 35 who has a family history of heart disease should have a checkup before doing any strenuous exercise to ensure that there are no signs of heart disease or high blood pressure. It should then be reasonably safe for you to exercise, as long as the exertion does not bring on any alarming symptoms.

COMBATING STRESS

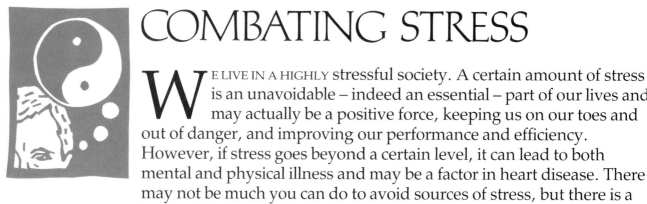

WE LIVE IN A HIGHLY stressful society. A certain amount of stress is an unavoidable – indeed an essential – part of our lives and may actually be a positive force, keeping us on our toes and out of danger, and improving our performance and efficiency. However, if stress goes beyond a certain level, it can lead to both mental and physical illness and may be a factor in heart disease. There may not be much you can do to avoid sources of stress, but there is a lot you can do to improve your ability to deal with it.

Most people believe that a high level of insecurity, anxiety, frequent crises, and constant conflicts play havoc with blood pressure and may eventually lead to a heart attack. In reality, although there is a strong link between persistently raised blood pressure and heart disease, links between stress and high blood pressure or heart disease are difficult to prove – partly because stress is so hard to define and quantify. It is thought, however, that certain people are more susceptible to heart disease than others due to their personalities.

Type B
The type B person is easygoing and relaxed, rarely in a hurry, neither competitive nor ambitious, finds it easy to delegate responsibility, and places less emphasis on work and career progression.

Type A
The type A person is impatient, highly competitive, aggressively ambitious, finds it difficult to delegate, has few interests outside the scope of his or her career or job performance, and often takes on many challenges simultaneously.

TYPES A AND B

A theory put forward in the 1960s claimed that there is a coronary-prone personality. This personality – defined by impatience and aggression – was called type A. The calmer, more relaxed personality was called type B. Studies of both personalities have shown that type A people are twice as likely to die of an initial heart attack as type B.

Changing your behavior
If you have a predominantly type A personality and wish to reduce your risk of heart trouble, you must acknowledge that you are indeed type A. Research shows that most type As deny this behavior pattern in themselves.

The second step is to believe in the ability to change this potentially harmful side of your nature. Many people succeed in doing this only after having a heart attack. How much better it would be to do it beforehand.

FIGHT OR FLIGHT

Our automatic reaction to any stressful situation is the "fight or flight" response. This primitive reflex prepares the body either to fight the enemy or to take flight by sending a message to the adrenal glands, which produce the hormones epinephrine and norepinephrine. These hormones manifest themselves in a

DEEP MUSCLE RELAXATION

Relaxation is a skill that needs to be learned and mastered. One of the simplest and most rewarding of these skills is deep muscle relaxation. Practice this routine slowly and thoroughly at least once a day, for 15 to 20 minutes. Always bring yourself out of relaxation gently, and do not practice on a full stomach.

2 Concentrate on relaxing each part of your body in turn. Concentrate first on your right foot and relax the toes, instep, heel, and ankle; feel the foot become totally relaxed and limp. Then move your attention up your leg, and relax the calf, knee, thigh, and hip. Do the same for your left leg.

4 Focus your attention on the base of your spine and relax your back muscles, working up the spine and the muscles on either side of it until you reach your neck.

1 Remove your shoes, any glasses or contact lenses, and any restrictive clothing. Lie flat on your back in a quiet, warm, dimly lit place. Let your feet flop outward, with your toes pointing outward. Allow your arms to fall away from your body, with your palms facing the ceiling and your fingers curling naturally. Breathe in and out gently, deeply, and at your own natural rhythm.

3 Next concentrate on your right hand and relax the fingers, thumb, palm, and wrist. Work slowly up the arm, relaxing your elbow, upper arm, and shoulder. Then focus your attention on your left hand and arm and do the same.

5 Finally, concentrate on your face. Relax your chin and jaw, making sure your tongue is relaxed. Focus on your eyes and forehead, and get rid of any frowns. Now you are completely relaxed. Concentrate on your breathing and, each time you exhale, let your body sink a little farther into the floor.

---

pounding, rapid heartbeat, rapid breathing, a dry mouth, gooseflesh, and an elevated blood pressure.

Back to normal

Once the threat or stressful situation is removed, the body returns to normal. If the source of stress is not removed, blood pressure may stay elevated for an indefinite period of time. This may be one factor in the development of coronary heart disease.

If you find you are frequently under stress and wish to protect your heart, three choices are open to you. You can seek ways of reducing stress levels, you can exercise more to release pent-up tension, or you can find methods of relaxing when the pressure is off. The DEEP MUSCLE RELAXATION box above details one type of relaxation exercise that you may find helpful.

FIVE METHODS TO REDUCE STRESS

♦ Create a more humane, evenly paced schedule for yourself, so that you are not under pressure constantly, either at work or when you are involved in an ostensibly relaxing activity.

♦ Take care of your personal life as well as your career. This entails developing interests that are not merely career-oriented. Perhaps the most significant of all is having satisfying relationships with other people.

♦ Exercise regularly to relieve stress, but try not to take your exercise too seriously. It is important to play games for enjoyment, not just to satisfy a compelling, competitive desire to win.

♦ Find time to practice the relaxation techniques of your choice. Listen to music, meditate, walk, or develop a hobby that pleasantly occupies you and makes you happy.

♦ A persistently stress-oriented approach to life may require a more profound investigation of the causes behind your stressful life patterns, perhaps with the aid of a psychiatrist.

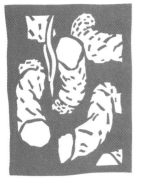

QUITTING SMOKING

MANY PEOPLE WHO are addicted to tobacco believe that smoking has no effect on the heart, but the evidence is loaded against them. The nicotine in tobacco smoke increases your heart rate and raises your blood pressure, while the carbon monoxide cuts down the amount of oxygen that can be carried by your blood. The heart must work harder but has less oxygen supplied to it. If you smoke, the best way to reduce your risk of heart disease is to quit.

WARNING

Cutting down on the number of cigarettes you smoke or switching to a low-tar or low-nicotine brand of cigarette is not as helpful as it might sound. Most people inhale more deeply to maintain their nicotine level.

Cigarette smokers who switch to a pipe or cigars often continue to inhale and probably do not decrease their risk substantially. They also risk getting oral and laryngeal cancers.

Everybody knows that smoking can cause lung cancer, but not everyone realizes how bad it is for the heart. Overall, cigarette smokers have a death rate from coronary heart disease that is 70 percent higher than that of nonsmokers. The more heavily you smoke, the greater the risk. If you smoke 40 or more cigarettes a day, you are between two and three times more likely to die of heart disease than a nonsmoker.

Smoking also increases the likelihood of cerebrovascular disease (disorders of blood vessels in the brain) and thus increases the risk of stroke (see page 121). It is also directly related to diseases of the arteries in the legs. Smokers make up at least 95 percent of patients suffering from these diseases – which can result in gangrene and amputation of the leg.

STOP NOW

A strong motivation to quit smoking is the most important factor in being successful. Some people find it easiest to go "cold turkey," quitting all smoking at once. Many people benefit from behavior modification programs.

If you give up smoking, your risk of heart disease declines rapidly. For example, if you consume less than one pack of cigarettes a day and give up now, after about 3 years of not smoking your risk of heart disease is almost identical to that of a lifelong nonsmoker. As the years without tobacco pass, the risk diminishes for other diseases as well. Every day spent without smoking is an investment in your future health.

THE SMOKING FACTOR

The bar chart at right shows how the mortality ratio (the number of times more likely an ex-smoker is of dying in any year than a lifelong nonsmoker) diminishes steadily with the number of years since quitting smoking.

Nonsmokers

Ex-smokers age 65+

Ex-smokers age 30 to 64

Mortality ratio

2.0
1.7
1.6
1.6
1.4
1.4
1.4
1.2
1.1
1.1

Less than 1   1 to 4   5 to 9   10 to 14   15+   Non-smokers

Years since smoking ceased

WHY DO YOU SMOKE?

To help you stop smoking, it is useful to think about your reasons for smoking and to decide what type of smoker you are. Answer these questions after careful consideration. Be honest in your assessment of your smoking habits. And remember – your desire to quit smoking is the most important and effective means of becoming an ex-smoker.

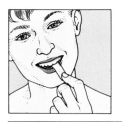

♦ **Do you smoke because you are truly addicted to nicotine?**
If so, you probably begin to feel restless and crave another cigarette a few minutes after finishing the previous one. You will do best with the "cold turkey" approach. Nicotine chewing gum, available by prescription, helps relieve withdrawal symptoms.

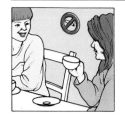

♦ **Do you smoke out of sheer habit or whenever you are unoccupied?**
You must break your habit pattern. Delay your first cigarette by an hour each day, smoke less of each cigarette, don't carry cigarettes, and sit in the "no-smoking" areas in restaurants and on airplanes. Also, try using your other hand to hold the cigarette.

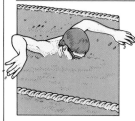

♦ **Do you smoke to help with tasks requiring mental concentration?**
If so, you probably have a problem with mental discipline. Physical exercise increases mental alertness and stamina and relieves depression, which will help you concentrate without cigarettes. In addition, it is difficult to smoke and exercise at the same time.

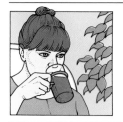

♦ **Do you smoke because you need something to do with your hands or mouth?**
Many smokers reach for a cigarette to alleviate boredom. You may need a hobby that keeps your hands occupied and is mentally stimulating in a nonstressful way. To keep your mouth occupied, try chewing on coffee stirrers, toothpicks, or gum.

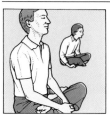

♦ **Do you smoke only when you are with other smokers?**
You may need to avoid socializing for a while with friends who smoke. This may seem to be a drastic measure, but consider it a short-term sacrifice that will add to the quality of your life. Once you have built up your resistance to the temptation to smoke, you can join them again.

♦ **Do you reach for your cigarettes as a way of relieving tension?**
In the long term, smoking can add to personal stress by impairing your health and thus your ability to cope with stress effectively. Learn some other ways of dealing with stressful situations, such as those detailed on page 29. Smoking doesn't solve any problems.

ASK YOUR DOCTOR
QUITTING SMOKING

Q I've smoked for more than 30 years. Is stopping really going to help my heart now?

A It's never too late. Studies show that ex-smokers are much less likely to have a heart attack than people who smoke. The risks associated with smoking decrease quickly in the first year of giving up.

Q My mother smoked 20 cigarettes a day all her life, and she died in her sleep when she was 92. Might I not be like her?

A There are always exceptions. In any case, your mother probably would have felt a lot healthier had she not smoked.

Q Is there any danger of becoming addicted to the nicotine chewing gum my doctor prescribed?

A Yes, but it's not as bad for you as smoking because you are not inhaling carbon particles and carbon monoxide from the cigarettes.

Q I'd like to quit smoking, but I worry about gaining weight. Isn't obesity just as bad for the heart?

A People do tend to put on weight when they quit smoking, but being overweight is not as bad for your heart as smoking. The average person gains only 5 to 10 pounds and some people don't gain any weight.

Q A friend of mine underwent hypnosis to help him stop smoking. Does hypnosis work?

A Some smokers find it helpful, but it works only if you are motivated to quit.

CHAPTER THREE

THE HEALTHY HEART

THE HEART ACTS as a pump. Its task is to maintain a constant circulation of blood around the body. These facts are familiar to us now, but, until the 17th century, doctors had no conception of blood circulation. They believed instead that blood was produced by the liver, after which it was dispatched just once by the heart to the body, where it lay static in reservoirs, until it was drained into the tissues to provide them with nourishment. When the body was punctured, the blood was perceived as simply pouring out of the reservoirs. Some doctors had an inkling of the truth of the matter. However, it was not always to their advantage. Michael Servetus (1511 - 1553), for example, was burned as a heretic in the 16th century for stating, correctly as it turns out, that blood passes from the right side of the heart to the left side via the

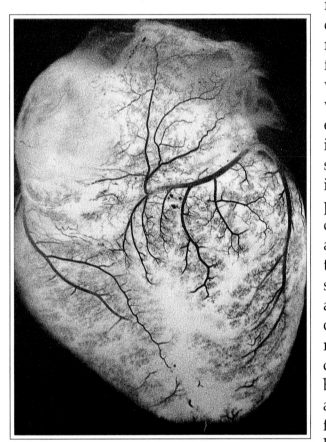

lungs. The years of confusion were finally laid to rest by the British physician William Harvey (1578-1657), who observed that the valves inside the heart permit blood only to flow away from the heart through certain blood vessels, while the valves inside veins allow blood only to return to the heart. From these observations, he deduced that blood must flow around the body in a continuous circuit.

In this chapter, the workings of the heart and the circulation are laid bare. The heart lies at the center of a network of blood vessels so vast that every living cell in the body is supplied with the oxygen and nutrients it needs. Subjected to the differing demands made by exercise or sleep, sexual intercourse or digestion, stress or relaxation, the heart faithfully responds by supplying just the right volume of blood needed to serve the occasion. To do so, it relies on the unique fibers of its hard-working muscular walls, on a complex electrical pacemaking and conducting system, on its own intricate blood supply provided by the coronary arteries, and on its vital internal valves, whose slamming shut against the pressure of blood causes the rhythmical "lubb-dupp" of the heartbeat. This chapter also explains the different phases of the heartbeat and the mechanisms by which the heart rate is controlled, the role that blood pressure plays in the circulatory system, and the way the heart automatically alters the blood pressure when stimulated. Your heart is indeed a complex organ. Appreciating the way it functions in its healthy state is the best starting point for a complete understanding of the different types of disorders to which it can fall prey.

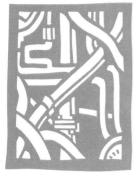

THE CIRCULATORY SYSTEM

AN ADEQUATE BLOOD CIRCULATION is essential for life and health. The blood is kept in constant circulation by the pumping action of the heart, which sends blood to the lungs to pick up oxygen, and then pumps it to the rest of the body. The blood is pushed through a system of tubes, which branch repeatedly into ever smaller and thinner-walled vessels, bringing life-sustaining blood into intimate contact with living cells throughout the body.

The heart and blood vessels act as a single system. But within it there are two distinct but linked circuits of blood vessels – the pulmonary circulation, which carries blood from the heart to the lungs and then back to the heart, and the systemic circulation, which distributes blood to all parts of the body and then returns it to the heart again. The average time it takes for blood to complete one full circuit of the system is 1 minute.

FUNCTION OF THE CIRCULATION

The circulation provides your body with a constant supply of oxygen, as well as fuel in the form of glucose, construction materials such as amino acids and cholesterol, and many other substances.

The first and most vital requirement is oxygen. Without oxygen, cells cease to

HOW THE BLOOD CIRCULATES

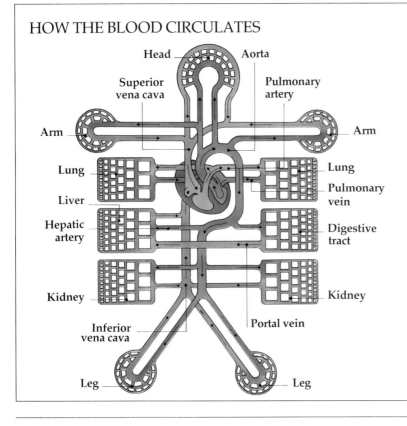

The heart is the center of the circulatory system. Deoxygenated (blue) blood flowing into the right side of the heart enters the pulmonary circulation. It is pumped via the pulmonary artery to the lungs, where it takes up oxygen. The oxygenated blood (red) is returned by the pulmonary veins to the left side of the heart, where it enters the systemic circulation. It is then pumped via the aorta to the head, arms, legs, and internal organs. There it passes through capillary networks, gives up its oxygen, and is returned via the venae cavae to the right side of the heart.

The liver receives two supplies of blood. The hepatic artery supplies oxygenated blood, while the portal vein transports blood from the intestines to the liver. The blood from the intestines is rich in the nutrient products of digestion, which are extracted by the liver before the blood is returned to the heart.

THE MAJOR BLOOD VESSELS

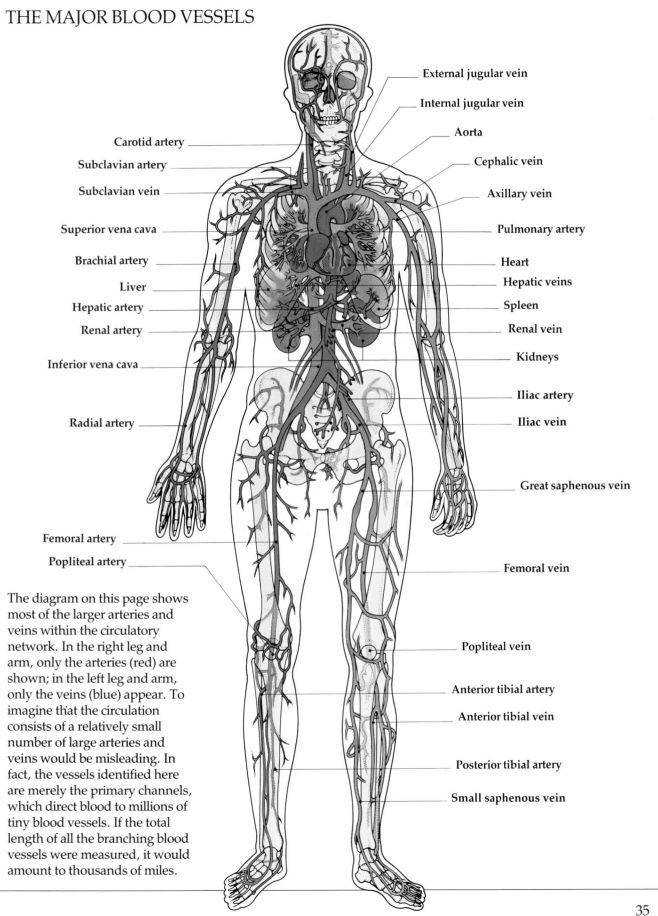

External jugular vein

Internal jugular vein

Aorta

Cephalic vein

Axillary vein

Pulmonary artery

Heart

Hepatic veins

Spleen

Renal vein

Kidneys

Iliac artery

Iliac vein

Great saphenous vein

Femoral vein

Popliteal vein

Anterior tibial artery

Anterior tibial vein

Posterior tibial artery

Small saphenous vein

Carotid artery

Subclavian artery

Subclavian vein

Superior vena cava

Brachial artery

Liver

Hepatic artery

Renal artery

Inferior vena cava

Radial artery

Femoral artery

Popliteal artery

The diagram on this page shows most of the larger arteries and veins within the circulatory network. In the right leg and arm, only the arteries (red) are shown; in the left leg and arm, only the veins (blue) appear. To imagine that the circulation consists of a relatively small number of large arteries and veins would be misleading. In fact, the vessels identified here are merely the primary channels, which direct blood to millions of tiny blood vessels. If the total length of all the branching blood vessels were measured, it would amount to thousands of miles.

function within a matter of minutes. Oxygen reaches the blood from air by way of the lungs. The blood must come into close contact with the air in the lungs before an adequate volume can pass into it. For this reason, the lungs also contain an intricate network of blood vessels.

The work of saturating the blood with oxygen is so important that it is the sole function of the pulmonary circulation, which is powered by its own pump, the right side of the heart. Once the blood has been oxygenated, it returns to the left side of the heart, from where it is pumped to the rest of the body.

Waste disposal

In addition to providing the transport medium for the cells' supplies, the blood in the systemic circulation carries unwanted waste material away from the tissues of the body. The waste gas, carbon dioxide, moves out of the tissues into the blood and is taken to the heart and then to the lungs, from where it is

exhaled. Other wastes are filtered and excreted into the urine by the kidneys, through which all the blood in the circulation passes many times a day.

THE BLOOD VESSELS

The heart forces blood under pressure through an extensive and intricate network of major and minor blood vessels. These vessels vary in character, depending on the demands that are made on them and the work they must do.

Arteries

The arteries carry blood away from the heart, either to the lungs (in the pulmonary circulation) or to the rest of the body. Arteries are thick-walled vessels that widen when blood is forced into them by the heart. They then contract automatically, pushing the blood onward through the circulatory system. The main arteries branch into small arteries (arterioles) and then into capillaries.

Capillary network
Between the smallest arteries (arterioles) and smallest veins (venules) in all the body tissues there exists a network of capillaries (below). The capillaries have a tiny diameter – just wide enough to allow the red blood cells to squeeze through. Each capillary has a very thin wall that contains tiny spaces. These spaces allow a fluid that contains oxygen and nutrients to move from the capillaries into the spaces between the cells of the surrounding tissue.

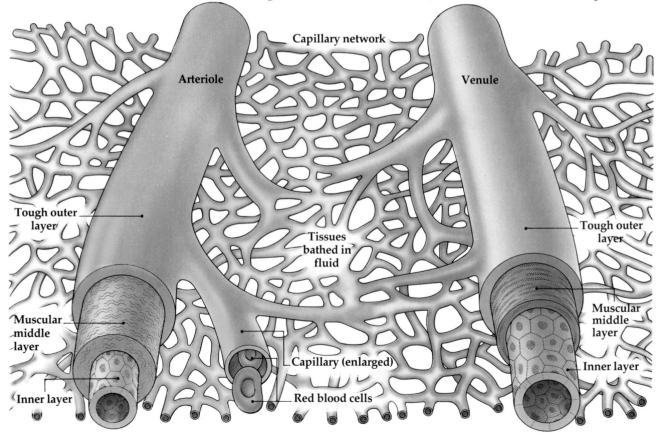

Veins

By the time the blood has passed through the arterioles into the capillaries, the pressure has dropped to almost zero. Because of this, the venules and veins, which carry blood back to the heart, are sometimes partially collapsed. Nevertheless, the volume of blood flowing through the venous and arterial systems is always equal.

Most of the veins contain valves that prevent backflow of blood (these are the valves that break down with varicose veins). All the systemic veins eventually carry blood back into two very large veins, called the venae cavae, which deliver the blood to the right side of the heart.

Movement of fluid

There is a continuous, dynamic movement of fluid between the capillaries and the cells that make up the surrounding tissues. The fluid containing oxygen and nutrients moves from the capillaries into the tissue fluid that bathes the body cells, but some tissue fluid containing waste products also moves back into the capillaries. The amount of fluid leaving the capillaries is a little greater than the amount entering them. The difference is returned to the circulation via the lymphatic drainage system (see below).

HOW DOES THE BLOOD CARRY OXYGEN?

Every drop of blood contains about 50 million red cells that are packed with the iron-containing pigment hemoglobin. Chemically, hemoglobin and oxygen link together readily. In any environment in which oxygen is plentiful (such as the lungs), the gas attaches itself to the hemoglobin to form the bright red compound oxyhemoglobin. The link between hemoglobin and oxygen is a loose one, however. When the hemoglobin moves into an environment of low oxygen content in the body tissues, it gives up its linked oxygen. The oxygen dissolves in the tissue fluids and is then picked up by the cells to be used in the production of energy.

Deoxygenated hemoglobin returning from the tissues is a dark purple-red. However, when this blood is pumped back to the lungs, the red cells are brought into close contact with oxygen contained in the lungs' air sacs. The hemoglobin in the blood immediately becomes fully saturated with oxygen and, as the red cells sweep back to the heart, they carry the life-sustaining oxygen with them.

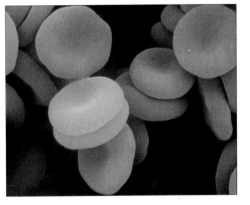

Red cells
The electron micrograph at left shows a number of red blood cells. Each cell contains hundreds of molecules of hemoglobin. The shape of the cells allows them to squeeze through the smallest blood vessels without being damaged.

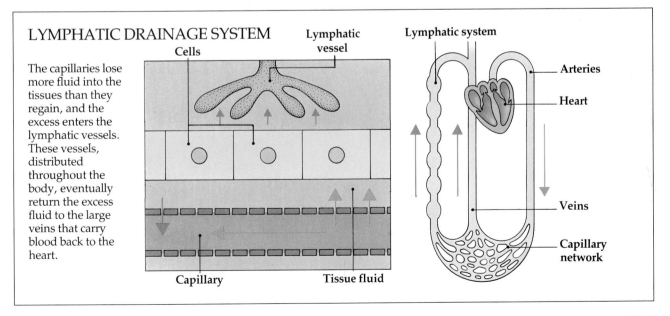

LYMPHATIC DRAINAGE SYSTEM

The capillaries lose more fluid into the tissues than they regain, and the excess enters the lymphatic vessels. These vessels, distributed throughout the body, eventually return the excess fluid to the large veins that carry blood back to the heart.

Cells

Lymphatic vessel

Capillary

Tissue fluid

Lymphatic system

Arteries

Heart

Veins

Capillary network

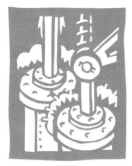

HOW YOUR HEART WORKS

THE HEART IS A HOLLOW, muscular organ situated just a little to the left of the center of the chest. It is slightly larger than a clenched fist and is the hardest-working muscle in your body. The range of demands you make on your heart varies widely under different conditions, depending on whether you are resting, walking leisurely, or exercising strenuously.

The heart works according to the pump principle. Imagine the inner tube of a bicycle tire filled with water. If you squeeze it, the water moves in both directions; when you release the tube, the water returns to its original position.

Now suppose there are valves inside the tube, shaped so that the water can move freely in only one direction. When

THE DUAL PUMP

Blood vessels connected to the heart carry blood to and from all parts of the body. "Used" blood from the body is returned to the heart and is pumped to the lungs, where it picks up oxygen; then it returns to the heart and is pumped throughout the body.

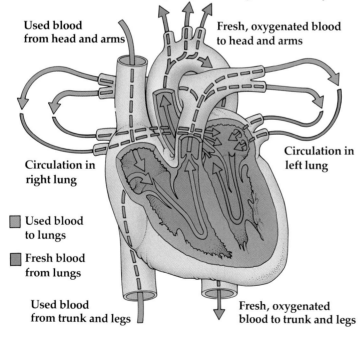

Used blood from head and arms

Fresh, oxygenated blood to head and arms

Circulation in right lung

Circulation in left lung

■ Used blood to lungs

■ Fresh blood from lungs

Used blood from trunk and legs

Fresh, oxygenated blood to trunk and legs

Superior vena cava

Right lung

Heart chambers
The heart is divided into four chambers – two thin-walled upper chambers, known as atria, and two thick-walled lower chambers, known as ventricles. The two sides of the heart are separated by a strong muscular wall known as the septum.

Right atrium

Pulmonary valve

Tricuspid valve

Heart muscle
The heart consists of a special type of muscle that is unique to the heart. Inside, the muscle fibers form a branching network. Given sufficient oxygen and nutrients, the heart muscle, also called the myocardium, contracts spontaneously, rhythmically, and automatically.

Chordae tendineae

Major blood vessels
The largest artery of the body, the aorta, leads from the left ventricle and supplies the body with oxygenated blood. The artery leading from the right ventricle is the pulmonary artery. The pulmonary artery divides into two branches that supply used blood to the right and left lungs.

Blood flow
The volume of blood pumped to the lungs by the right ventricle must be the same as the volume pumped by the left ventricle. But the resistance to blood flow through the general circulation is much greater than the resistance to flow through the lungs, so the left side of the heart must contract more forcibly. The muscle wall on the left side of the heart is consequently thicker and stronger.

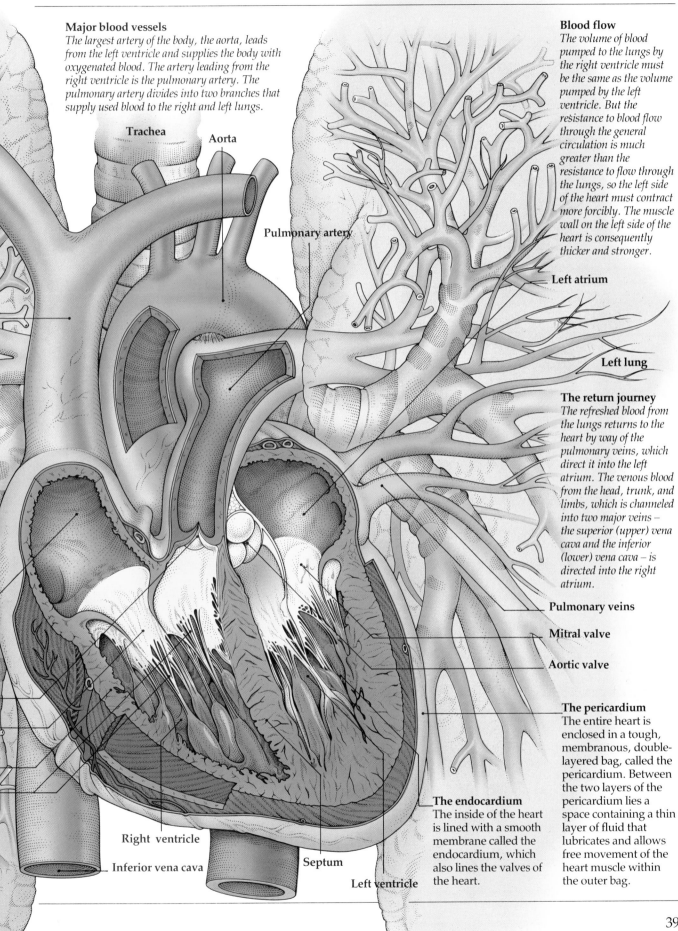

Trachea

Aorta

Pulmonary artery

Left atrium

Left lung

The return journey
The refreshed blood from the lungs returns to the heart by way of the pulmonary veins, which direct it into the left atrium. The venous blood from the head, trunk, and limbs, which is channeled into two major veins – the superior (upper) vena cava and the inferior (lower) vena cava – is directed into the right atrium.

Pulmonary veins

Mitral valve

Aortic valve

The pericardium
The entire heart is enclosed in a tough, membranous, double-layered bag, called the pericardium. Between the two layers of the pericardium lies a space containing a thin layer of fluid that lubricates and allows free movement of the heart muscle within the outer bag.

The endocardium
The inside of the heart is lined with a smooth membrane called the endocardium, which also lines the valves of the heart.

Right ventricle

Inferior vena cava

Septum

Left ventricle

the water tries to move in the opposite direction, the valves close.

If you squeeze anywhere on the tube, the entire volume of water will move in one direction. If you squeeze regularly, the water will circulate for as long as the squeezing continues. The function of the heart is to supply the regular squeezing that forces blood around the circulatory system. The heart contains valves so the blood can move in one direction only.

THE HEARTBEAT SEQUENCE

The heartbeat sequence has three phases. The timing of the phases must be accurately maintained, regardless of how slowly or rapidly the heart is beating. The rhythm is achieved by electrical impulses that come from the heart's pacemaker, the sinoatrial node. This node is made up of a group of nerve cells in the wall of the right atrium.

Diastole

During the first phase in the heartbeat sequence, called diastole, the heart fills with blood. At the same time, blood ejected from the heart during the previous contraction has time to move away. During most of diastole, blood flows into the atria (the upper heart chambers) and through the valves at the exits of the atria into the ventricles (the lower heart chambers). The ventricles fill because they actively dilate (open up) during diastole so they are at a lower pressure than the atria. By the end of diastole, the ventricles are filled to about 80 percent capacity.

Atrial systole

The next phase in the heartbeat sequence is called atrial systole. During this phase, the atria contract to squeeze the remainder of the blood they contain into the ventricles. Atrial systole is initiated by an

THE CORONARY SYSTEM

Because the heart is the hardest-working muscle in the body, it has large energy requirements. Like all other muscles, it requires an adequate supply of fresh, oxygenated blood to maintain its action. The blood that passes through the heart as part of the general circulatory system cannot provide the necessary supply because it does not have the intricate, intimate access to the muscle cells deep within the heart wall.

The heart therefore has its own system of arteries, capillaries, and veins exclusively for its own requirements. This is the coronary system, so named because the arteries surround the upper part of the heart like a crown ("corona" being the Latin word for crown).

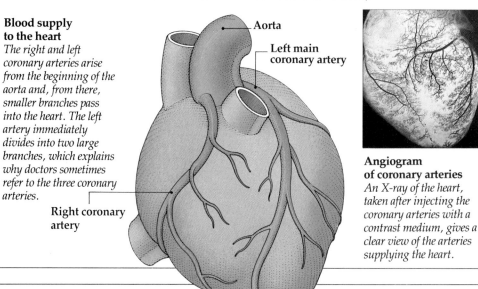

Blood supply to the heart
The right and left coronary arteries arise from the beginning of the aorta and, from there, smaller branches pass into the heart. The left artery immediately divides into two large branches, which explains why doctors sometimes refer to the three coronary arteries.

Aorta

Left main coronary artery

Right coronary artery

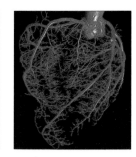

Angiogram of coronary arteries
An X-ray of the heart, taken after injecting the coronary arteries with a contrast medium, gives a clear view of the arteries supplying the heart.

Resin cast of coronary arteries
This resin cast shows the arrangement of the coronary arteries and their branches, which supply blood and oxygen to the heart muscle.

HOW THE HEART VALVES WORK

The heart valves ensure that blood flows through the heart in one direction only. Defective heart valves are the cause of several disorders.

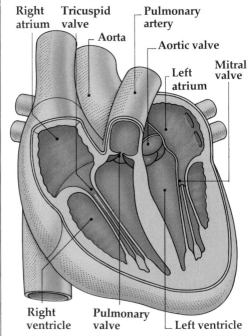

Right atrium
Tricuspid valve
Aorta
Pulmonary artery
Aortic valve
Mitral valve
Left atrium
Right ventricle
Pulmonary valve
Left ventricle

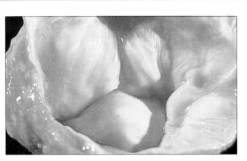

The heart valves
The pulmonary and aortic valves guard the opening of the right ventricle into the pulmonary artery and the opening of the left ventricle into the aorta. The valves are made up of three cusps that flip open when blood is forced through them, but fit together tightly when closed. The larger mitral and tricuspid valves permit blood to flow from atrium to ventricle but not from ventricle to atrium.

Pulmonary valve
The pulmonary valve controls the blood flowing out of the heart and into the pulmonary artery. Like the aortic and tricuspid valves, it has three cusps; the mitral is the only bicuspid heart valve.

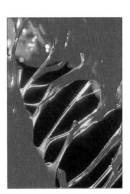

Chordae tendineae
To prevent the tricuspid and mitral valves from being forced upward by the pressure of blood, these valves are fastened to the ventricular walls with fibrous strands called chordae tendineae.

electrical impulse from the sinoatrial node that spreads over the atria, causing them to contract.

Ventricular systole

At the end of atrial systole, the electrical impulse from the sinoatrial node reaches a second node, called the atrioventricular node, situated at the junction between the atria and the ventricles. After a slight delay, the impulse then spreads from the atrioventricular node to the ventricles. This leads to the third phase of the heartbeat sequence, called ventricular systole, during which the ventricles contract. As the ventricles begin to contract, the pressure in them exceeds the pressure in the atria, and the valves between the ventricles and atria close tightly. Shortly afterward, the valves at the exits from the ventricles open, and blood is forced out of the heart into the pulmonary artery and the aorta, causing a steep rise in pressure in both these arteries.

At the end of ventricular systole, diastole begins again. The valves at the exits from the ventricles close to prevent blood from flowing back into the heart from the arteries. The valves between the atria and ventricles open up again as the heart begins to refill with blood.

CARDIAC OUTPUT

An important measure of the efficiency of the heart is the cardiac output. Also called the stroke volume, cardiac output is the volume of blood pumped by each contraction multiplied by the number of contractions, or beats, per minute. If, for instance, each ventricle ejects 2 ounces (62 milliliters) of blood per beat and the heart rate is 72 beats per minute, the cardiac output is 72 x 2 ounces (62 milliliters) or 9 pints (4.5 liters) per minute.

The rate at which the heart beats and the amount of blood it pushes out with each contraction can vary widely accord-

HEART FACTS

◆ The heart beats about 70 times a minute at rest.

◆ It can beat up to 200 times a minute during strenuous exercise.

◆ The heart contracts about 100,000 times every day and more than 2.5 billion times in an average lifetime.

◆ It pumps at least 9 pints (4.5 liters) of blood per minute.

◆ It pumps about 1,500 gallons (6,000 liters) of blood every day.

◆ The heart generates enough power in a day to drive a truck 20 miles.

CONTROL OF THE HEARTBEAT

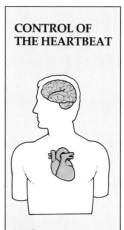

100 beats per minute
In the absence of nervous system control, the heart would beat at about 100 impulses per minute.

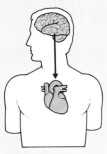

70 beats per minute
At rest, the heart rate is kept slower by parasympathetic nerves, especially the vagus nerve.

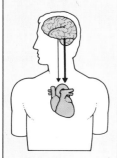

140 beats per minute
During exercise, parasympathetic activity lessens and the sympathetic nervous system speeds up the heart rate.

HOW YOUR HEART BEATS

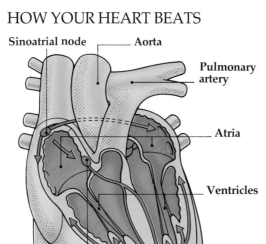

Sinoatrial node — Aorta

Pulmonary artery

Atria

Ventricles

Atrioventricular node

Electrical impulses
The timing of the heartbeat is kept by electrical impulses that are controlled by the sinoatrial node, the body's natural pacemaker. The pause between atrial and ventricular contractions is controlled by a second node, called the atrioventricular node.

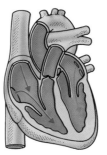
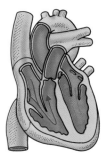

Diastole
During this resting phase, the heart fills with blood. Deoxygenated blood flows into the right side and oxygenated blood flows into the left side.

Atrial systole
In the second phase, the two atria contract simultaneously, squeezing more blood into the two ventricles, which become fully filled.

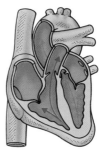

Ventricular systole
The ventricles contract to pump deoxygenated blood into the pulmonary artery and oxygenated blood into the aorta. When the heart is emptied, diastole begins again.

ing to the level of exertion. As the muscles use up oxygen and fuel, an increased demand is made on the heart for more blood. During strenuous exercise, the heart rate may increase to 200 beats per minute and the stroke volume may increase to more than twice its resting figure, raising the total output to about 54 pints (27 liters) per minute.

Changes in rate and output

Changes in rate and output are brought about in two ways. First, any increase in the amount of blood returning to the heart results in increased filling of the ventricles, which stretch to accommodate the greater volume of blood. When the ventricles are stretched in this way, the force of their contraction increases and, as a result, the stroke volume increases correspondingly.

Second, the heart rate is under the external control of the sympathetic and parasympathetic nervous systems, which can, respectively, accelerate or decelerate the heart rate.

CONTROL OF THE HEART RATE

The autonomic nervous system is the part of the nervous system concerned with unconscious, automatic control of many body functions. The autonomic nervous system is divided into the sympathetic and the parasympathetic branches, which oppose each other.

Sympathetic and parasympathetic activity

Sympathetic nerve stimulation speeds up the heart, while parasympathetic stimulation slows it down. At rest, the parasympathetic nerves (especially the vagus nerve) exert the greatest control. The signals carried by the vagus nerve act on the sinoatrial node to slow the heart rate from about 100 impulses per minute to a rate closer to 70 per minute. This action is known as vagal inhibition. During exertion, vagal inhibition lessens, and the heart rate speeds up.

When there is a need for a greater cardiac output, the sympathetic nervous system comes into action. First, the rate is speeded up by the direct action of nerve impulses on the heart. Second, the adrenal glands release the hormones epinephrine and norepinephrine. These hormones help speed the heart rate, raise the blood pressure, and constrict the blood vessels in the skin and digestive system, diverting the blood to the muscles and preparing the body for physical action. This combination of nervous and hormonal control allows the cardiovascular system to respond to stress in two ways – an immediate, nervous response and a more delayed, sustained hormonal reaction.

It is interesting to note that the heart can respond to the demands of exercise even if its nerve supply is completely cut off. This is partly due to the release of hormones by the adrenal glands.

EXERCISE AND THE HEALTHY HEART

Because of the sensitive way in which the heart responds to bodily demands, exercising any part of the body also exercises the heart. Exercise increases the efficiency of contraction and output of the heart per beat. Conversely, because the demand on heart output (blood pumped per minute) remains constant in a person at rest, so the heart rate needed to maintain this output is less in a physically fit person. A regular exercise program can actually reduce the resting pulse rate. Athletes who are in top condition may have a resting pulse rate of as low as 40 beats per minute.

In addition, because of the increase in blood output per heartbeat in a physically fit person, the heart does not have to beat as fast during any form of exercise.

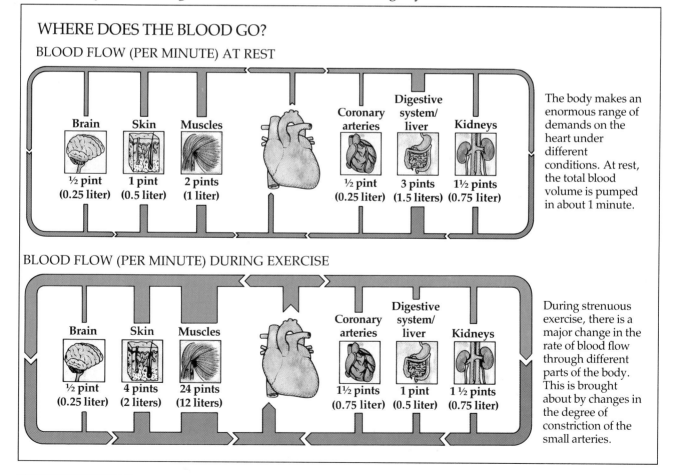

WHERE DOES THE BLOOD GO?

BLOOD FLOW (PER MINUTE) AT REST

Brain	Skin	Muscles		Coronary arteries	Digestive system/liver	Kidneys
½ pint (0.25 liter)	1 pint (0.5 liter)	2 pints (1 liter)		½ pint (0.25 liter)	3 pints (1.5 liters)	1½ pints (0.75 liter)

The body makes an enormous range of demands on the heart under different conditions. At rest, the total blood volume is pumped in about 1 minute.

BLOOD FLOW (PER MINUTE) DURING EXERCISE

Brain	Skin	Muscles		Coronary arteries	Digestive system/liver	Kidneys
½ pint (0.25 liter)	4 pints (2 liters)	24 pints (12 liters)		1½ pints (0.75 liter)	1 pint (0.5 liter)	1½ pints (0.75 liter)

During strenuous exercise, there is a major change in the rate of blood flow through different parts of the body. This is brought about by changes in the degree of constriction of the small arteries.

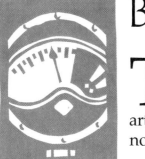

BLOOD PRESSURE

THE BLOOD IN YOUR ARTERIES must be kept at a certain pressure to maintain your circulation. This pressure varies with the output of blood from your heart and the resistance of the smallest arteries to blood flow. In a healthy person, the blood pressure normally remains within strict limits.

The pressure inside any system filled with fluid – such as the circulatory system – depends on the volume of fluid in it and how easily the walls can be stretched. If the walls are highly elastic, large quantities of fluid can be pushed through without much rise in pressure. However, if the walls are rigid and resist stretching, the addition of a very small amount of fluid causes a sharp rise in pressure. These facts are highly relevant to the heart and circulation.

WHAT INFLUENCES BLOOD PRESSURE?

Two factors act to raise blood pressure – any increase in the rate at which blood is pumped from the heart into the circulation (heart output) and any increase in the resistance of the arteries to the flow of blood.

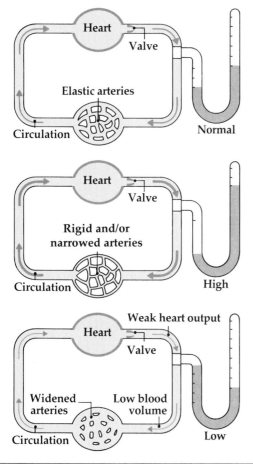

Normal
When healthy, the small arteries are elastic, and many of them expand during exercise. These factors level out changes in blood pressure as heart output rises and falls during rest and exercise.

High
High blood pressure may be persistently raised if the resistance of the circulation to blood flow increases because the small arteries are narrowed or have lost their elasticity due to disease.

Low
Blood pressure may drop dangerously if heart output falls due to a serious heart abnormality, if the blood volume falls due to serious bleeding, or if the small arteries widen, as they do in shock.

BLOOD PRESSURE VARIATIONS

Because the heart pumps in pulses, the blood pressure in the arteries is constantly changing, even at rest. It rises to a peak (the systolic pressure) during the contraction of the heart's ventricles and drops to a minimum level (the diastolic pressure) between beats.

Healthy arteries are elastic and "give" easily as blood is pumped into them. In addition, healthy arteries are totally clear with no abnormal narrowing or obstruction. This means that they are able to cope with the surge of blood that occurs with each heartbeat. It also means that the difference between diastolic and systolic pressures is not great.

High blood pressure
In some people the resistance of the smallest arteries to blood flow increases, often because of disease that causes the arteries to become rigid or narrowed. This leads to persistently raised levels of the diastolic or systolic blood pressure, or to a large difference between the two, even at rest. Persistently high blood pressure tends to cause the kind of damage to the arteries, such as loss of elasticity and narrowing, that in turn leads to still higher blood pressure.

MEASURING BLOOD PRESSURE

Measuring blood pressure is a simple procedure using a device called a sphygmomanometer. The pressure in the artery of the upper arm – the brachial artery – is measured using a cuff around the upper arm that is connected to a pressure-measuring device.

The reading

Because the earliest sphygmomanometers used a mercury column calibrated against a millimeter scale, blood pressure is recorded in millimeters of mercury (mm Hg). It is normal for blood pressure to rise as you get older. But anyone with a systolic pressure below 150 mm Hg and a diastolic pressure below 90 mm Hg is considered to have normal blood pressure. Most young people have a blood pressure of 130/80 mm Hg or less.

BLOOD PRESSURE AND EXERCISE

During exercise, blood flow to the muscles increases. This requires an increase in the heart's output of blood, which would be expected to drive up the blood pressure. However, the increase in heart output is accompanied by some widening of the blood vessels that supply the muscles used during exercise. As a result, the resistance to blood flow is lessened considerably. During most exercise, the heart output increases more than the resistance decreases, resulting in a slight increase in the diastolic blood pressure. However, because the force of the heart's contractions increases greatly during vigorous exercise, the peaks of pressure tend to be far higher than normal, increasing the systolic pressure. This elevated pressure response is normal, and causes no harm.

SYSTOLE AND DIASTOLE

Unlike an electric water pump, which does its work continuously, the heart's pumping action is cyclical in nature. It rhythmically beats and then relaxes, creating a varying pressure wave (see right). When the heart relaxes between beats, and the ventricles fill with blood from the atria, arterial blood pressure is at its lowest (known as the diastolic pressure). The ventricles then contract forcefully, increasing the arterial blood pressure until it reaches its peak elevation (known as the systolic pressure).

The increase in the pressure during systole is due partly to the strength of the contraction needed to force out the volume of blood from the ventricles when the heart contracts, and partly to the elastic recoil produced by the stretched blood vessels. These vessels are most elastic in younger people. Their flexibility under the force of pressure from the heart holds down the pressure wave and helps keep blood pressure low.

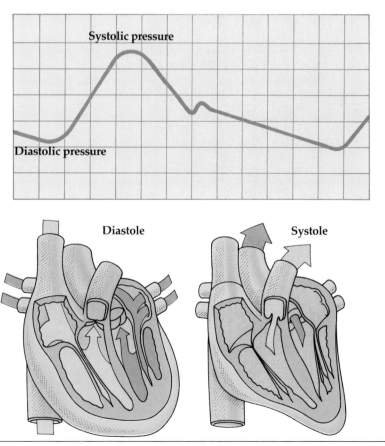

Systolic pressure

Diastolic pressure

Diastole

Systole

CHAPTER FOUR

INVESTIGATING HEART DISEASE

WHEN SYMPTOMS of a heart or circulatory disorder develop today, doctors are better equipped than ever before to find out what is wrong. This chapter reviews the techniques and equipment that cardiologists and other doctors use to diagnose cardiovascular disease. The chapter begins with a familiar type of investigation – listening to the heart through a stethoscope. Although this might appear to be a relatively simple procedure, in practice it requires years of experience – with hours and hours of listening time – to distinguish the various types of murmurs, clicks, snaps, rumbles, and other abnormal sounds that can indicate a disorder of the heart. Electrocardiography, covered in the next section, is probably the most frequently used test for evaluating the status of the heart. With its refinements, such as exercise electrocardiography and ambulatory electrocardiography, it is used universally for assessing all types of heart rate and rhythm disturbances, heart muscle damage from coronary heart disease, and many other types of heart disorders. This section reviews not only how the various types of electrocardiograms (ECGs) are carried out, but also what an ECG tracing can reveal about heart function or dysfunction.

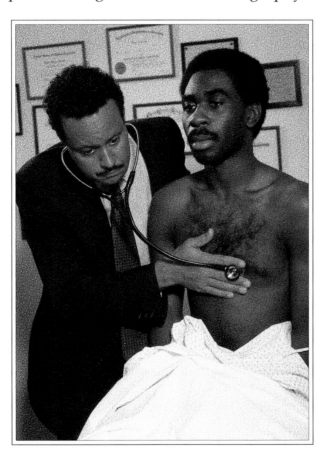

For imaging the heart and blood vessels, today's cardiologist has a wide variety of techniques at his or her disposal. Some of these procedures produce frontal views of the heart; others produce cross-sectional or even three-dimensional images, or video recordings showing blood flow through the heart and blood vessels. Some of the techniques, such as chest X-rays and echocardiography, are most useful for revealing abnormalities of size, structure, or anatomy. Others, such as Doppler scanning and the various types of radionuclide scans, can reveal abnormalities of function as well. These techniques, their uses, and what it feels like to have them performed are covered in a special section of the chapter. The final sections explain cardiac catheterization and the tests on blood and other body fluids that are used for diagnosing heart disease. Cardiac catheterization is a slightly risky procedure that is nevertheless necessary to obtain vital anatomic information about the heart and coronary arteries before surgery. Blood tests are highly important in assessing the severity of damage after a heart attack, and in gauging the body's response to treatment. The choice of tests depends on the doctor's interpretation of a disorder, and on the information he or she needs.

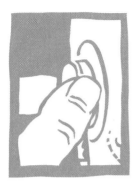

LISTENING TO THE HEART

T HE FAMILIAR AND REASSURING sound of the heartbeat is made by the opening and closing of the four valves that control the circulation of blood through the heart. Your doctor uses a stethoscope to hear the sounds of the heart more clearly. By listening closely, he or she can learn a great deal about the condition of your heart. However, heart sounds cannot reveal coronary heart disease.

Examining with a stethoscope
Your doctor will place the end of the stethoscope onto four different sites on the front of your chest. These sites correspond to the position of each of your four heart valves. You may be asked to lie on your left side or to sit leaning forward. You may also be asked to hold your breath for a few seconds so that the heart sounds are not muffled by the sounds of your lungs.

The standard stethoscope consists of a Y-shaped flexible plastic tube with an earpiece at the end of each arm of the Y and a sound-amplifying device attached to the base. This device has a thin, plastic diaphragm on one side and a concave bell with a small hole in its center on the other. The diaphragm is used to pick up high-pitched sounds and is pressed firmly against the chest wall. The bell is used to amplify quieter, deeper sounds and is placed gently against your skin.

HEART SOUNDS

There are two normal sounds made by the heart each time it beats. The first sound is heard as a "lubb" and is caused by the tricuspid and mitral valves slamming shut. The second is a more high-pitched "dupp;" it results from the closing of the pulmonary and aortic valves. The second sound is often split into a double sound, especially in children and young adults, because the aortic and pulmonary valves are not closing at the same time. This slight delay is very common and does not affect the heart's pumping mechanism.

Abnormal heart sounds
A heart disorder, such as a damaged valve, may signal itself by an abnormal sound such as a snap, click, or murmur or by an additional sound that is not normally present.

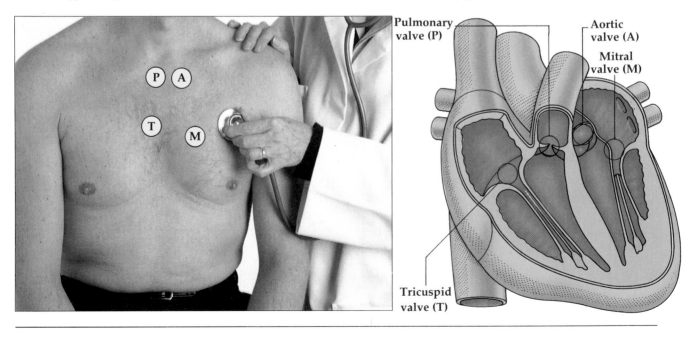

Pulmonary valve (P)

Aortic valve (A)

Mitral valve (M)

Tricuspid valve (T)

MURMURS CAUSED BY VALVE DISORDERS

Although the flow of blood in the heart is usually almost inaudible, turbulence of blood within the heart can create the sounds known as murmurs. Defective valves are a common cause. In stenosis, for example, the flaps of the valve fail to open wide enough, and sound is created by blood rushing around and behind them. An incompetent valve fails to close properly, and audible turbulence is caused by the collision of blood flowing under pressure from opposite directions.

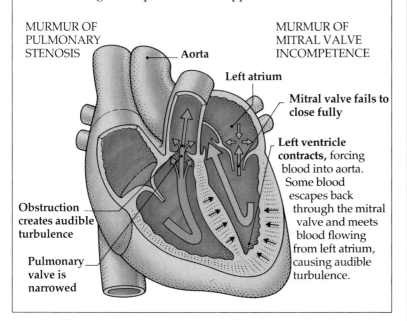

MURMUR OF PULMONARY STENOSIS

MURMUR OF MITRAL VALVE INCOMPETENCE

Aorta

Left atrium

Mitral valve fails to close fully

Left ventricle contracts, forcing blood into aorta. Some blood escapes back through the mitral valve and meets blood flowing from left atrium, causing audible turbulence.

Obstruction creates audible turbulence

Pulmonary valve is narrowed

Additional heart sounds include a third sound that occurs soon after the second. Although this sound is considered normal in young people, it is usually a sign of heart failure in anyone over age 40. A fourth heart sound, occurring as a low-pitched noise just before the first sound, indicates abnormal filling of the upper chambers of the heart. It sometimes occurs after a heart attack, or in a person who is suffering from a disease of the heart muscle.

A murmur is a whooshing noise heard between the normal heart sounds and is the result of turbulent blood flow. This turbulence may be caused by a damaged heart valve or by a congenital heart defect. Not all murmurs are due to a structural abnormality in the heart. Excessive turbulence of blood flow occasionally occurs through a normal heart valve, especially in young people.

SNAPS AND CLICKS

These sounds are heard through the stethoscope. An opening snap, heard shortly after the second heart sound, occurs when an abnormally narrow mitral valve opens.

High blood pressure and a variety of heart valve defects may cause one of the valves to click. The click is caused by abrupt halting of the opening of the valve.

ASK YOUR DOCTOR HEART SOUNDS

Q **Our daughter has just had her first child, and we are worried because our little grandson has been diagnosed with a heart murmur. Does this mean that there is something seriously wrong with his heart?**

A Many babies are born with a murmur, which in many cases disappears within a few days. Even if the murmur persists, the heart may be perfectly healthy. The doctors will probably check your grandson's heart and blood pressure again and, if necessary, will arrange for more tests such as echocardiography (see page 55) to find out whether there is any defect that requires surgery.

Q **If someone has a heart valve disorder, can a doctor tell exactly what is wrong just by listening to the way it sounds?**

A The characteristics of an abnormal heart sound, such as a murmur, and its location can help identify which valve is malfunctioning. The timing of a murmur – that is, whether it occurs during the heartbeat (systole) or between heartbeats (diastole) – determines whether the valve is opening and closing effectively. The murmur's loudness can reflect the severity of the damage. Although all these factors provide clues, more tests (such as echocardiography) may be needed to confirm the diagnosis.

Q **Can listening to the heart be used to predict whether a person is at risk of a heart attack?**

A No. Some heart disorders, such as coronary heart disease, usually have no effect on the heart sounds. Other tests are needed to make the diagnosis.

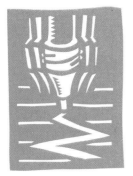

ELECTRO-CARDIOGRAPHY

I F YOU HAVE A HEART DISORDER, or your doctor suspects that you have one, you will probably require an electrocardiographic examination. This safe and painless test detects the flow of electricity through the heart immediately prior to each heartbeat via conducting plates (electrodes) attached to the skin. The pattern of electrical impulses is recorded on a moving strip of paper or on a monitor to produce an image known as an electrocardiogram (ECG).

In a healthy person, the passage of electrical impulses through the heart follows a regular, characteristic sequence. If there is any abnormality, this pattern is altered. Different abnormalities produce different patterns, allowing the doctor to diagnose a wide range of disorders.

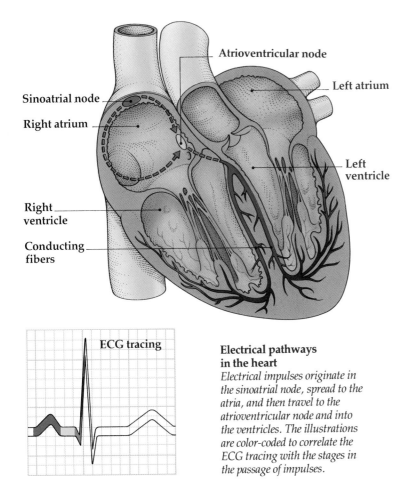

Electrical pathways in the heart
Electrical impulses originate in the sinoatrial node, spread to the atria, and then travel to the atrioventricular node and into the ventricles. The illustrations are color-coded to correlate the ECG tracing with the stages in the passage of impulses.

HOW DOES ELECTRO-CARDIOGRAPHY WORK?

Each heartbeat is brought about by electrical impulses that originate at the top of the heart in the sinoatrial node. The impulses spread through the atria to another node, the atrioventricular node, and then pass through the powerful lower pumping chambers (ventricles) via special conducting muscle fibers.

Because the body consists largely of salty water, which is an excellent conductor of electricity, the electrical changes in the heart also cause changes throughout the body that can be detected on its surface by electrodes. The electrodes are connected by wires to a meter (the ECG machine) that amplifies the electrical impulses and either records them on paper by a pen attached to the meter or displays them on a monitor.

During an ECG, electrodes are connected to the two wrists and the ankles (the right ankle serving as a ground) and to six different points on the chest. However, only two electrodes are activated at any time to make a complete circuit. Each circuit is known as a lead. There are 12 standard leads, each of which "looks" at a slightly different part of the heart. In this way, an ECG enables the doctor to locate the actual site of any damage to the heart muscle.

RECORDING AN ECG

To make an ECG recording, two electrodes at a time are activated to make a complete circuit (called a lead) with the ECG machine. The ECG recording from each lead reflects activity from a different part of the heart and, accordingly, each looks slightly different. For the chest leads, one input consists of three limb electrodes joined together and the other is taken from each of a series of six positions on the chest.

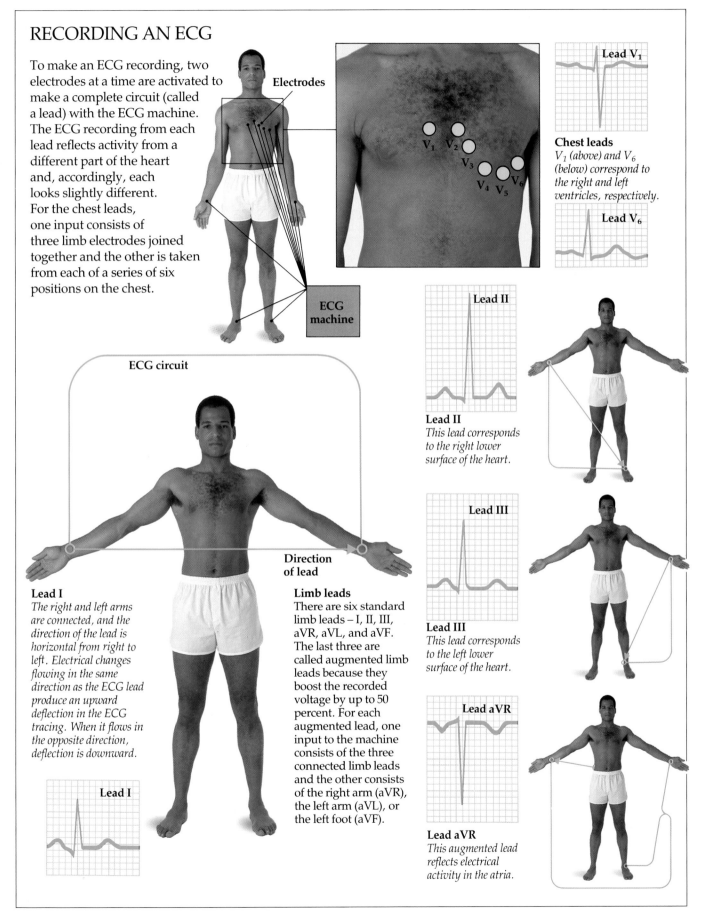

Electrodes

V_1 V_2 V_3 V_4 V_5 V_6

ECG machine

Lead V_1

Chest leads
V_1 (above) and V_6 (below) correspond to the right and left ventricles, respectively.

Lead V_6

ECG circuit

Direction of lead

Lead I
The right and left arms are connected, and the direction of the lead is horizontal from right to left. Electrical changes flowing in the same direction as the ECG lead produce an upward deflection in the ECG tracing. When it flows in the opposite direction, deflection is downward.

Lead I

Limb leads
There are six standard limb leads – I, II, III, aVR, aVL, and aVF. The last three are called augmented limb leads because they boost the recorded voltage by up to 50 percent. For each augmented lead, one input to the machine consists of the three connected limb leads and the other consists of the right arm (aVR), the left arm (aVL), or the left foot (aVF).

Lead II

Lead II
This lead corresponds to the right lower surface of the heart.

Lead III

Lead III
This lead corresponds to the left lower surface of the heart.

Lead aVR

Lead aVR
This augmented lead reflects electrical activity in the atria.

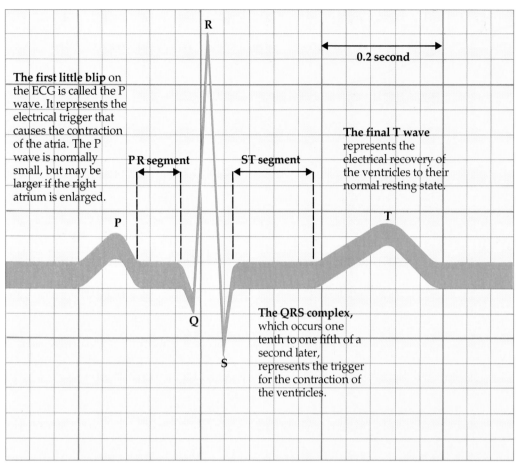

R

0.2 second

The first little blip on the ECG is called the P wave. It represents the electrical trigger that causes the contraction of the atria. The P wave is normally small, but may be larger if the right atrium is enlarged.

P R segment

ST segment

The final T wave represents the electrical recovery of the ventricles to their normal resting state.

P

T

Q

S

The QRS complex, which occurs one tenth to one fifth of a second later, represents the trigger for the contraction of the ventricles.

Interpreting an ECG
This diagram of an ECG of a normal heart shows the general features common to all leads. Because the ventricular, or lower, part of the heart contains many more muscle fibers than the atrial, or upper, part, the QRS complex (near the center of the diagram) is much more conspicuous than the P wave. The rising R deflection represents positive voltage, and the falling S deflection a negative voltage. Whereas the electrical recovery of the ventricles is marked by the T wave, the recovery of the atria is masked by the QRS complex and is not seen.

In a healthy person, the P and T waves are fairly constant in different lead recordings, but the QRS complex varies considerably from one lead recording to another.

USES OF THE ECG

An ECG helps the doctor investigate and diagnose a wide range of heart disorders. It is most commonly used to analyze abnormal heart rhythms, to identify defects in the conduction of electrical impulses through the heart, to identify areas of heart muscle that have been damaged by coronary heart disease, and to detect thickening of the walls of the heart muscle.

The fact that each lead reflects the activity in a slightly different portion of the heart means that the doctor is able to identify the specific area within the heart that is causing the problem.

Another use of the ECG is to test the function of an implanted pacemaker. The doctor holds a magnet about 1 inch from the pacemaker site while recording an ECG tracing. If the pacemaker is functioning normally, the magnet causes it to fire regularly. ECGs may also be performed periodically during drug treatment for heart disorders to check on the effectiveness of the treatment.

Continuous monitoring

In most cases, an ECG is performed while you are lying down. However, to detect disorders in which abnormal heart activity occurs intermittently, continuous monitoring for 24 to 48 hours is required. This is done by using a portable device, called a Holter monitor, that you wear while you go on with your normal daily activities. The monitor incorporates an amplifier and cassette tape on which the heart's electrical impulses are recorded. The patient keeps track of the exact times of changes in activities or emotional states so that they can later be interpreted and related to any changes on the ECG.

Heart attack

Within the first few hours of a heart attack, the ECG may be virtually normal. Damage to the heart muscle then causes changes in the QRS complex, the T wave, and the ST segment.

After a few hours, an abnormally deep Q deflection may appear and the ST segment is raised above the baseline. After a few days, the T wave becomes inverted (ECG at right). As the heart heals, these waves return to normal. If there is any substantial permanent damage to the muscular wall, the Q wave persists (ECG at far right).

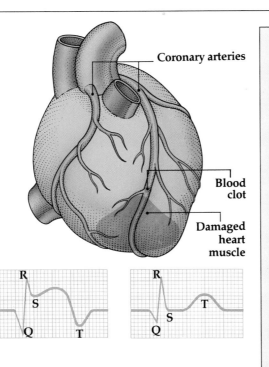

Coronary arteries

Blood clot

Damaged heart muscle

Enlargement of left ventricle

The left ventricle becomes enlarged if it must work harder for any reason, such as increased resistance due to high blood pressure. An enlarged left ventricle is characterized on an ECG tracing by an increase in the size of the S wave in the right chest lead (V_1) and an increase in the R wave in the left chest leads (V_2 to V_6).

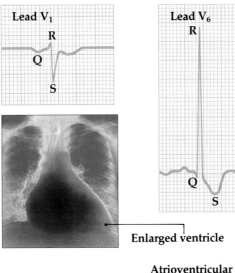

Lead V_1

Lead V_6

Enlarged ventricle

Ventricular fibrillation

In this type of abnormal heart rhythm, the ventricles beat extremely rapidly. The ECG shows no distinct QRS complexes, merely irregular rapid undulations, which may be of relatively high amplitude (coarse) or relatively low amplitude (fine), as shown below. The condition produces no effective heart pumping and is fatal within a few minutes unless treated.

Atrioventricular node

Sinoatrial node

Chaotic ventricular activity

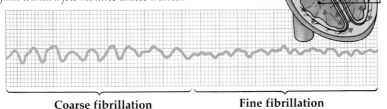

Coarse fibrillation   Fine fibrillation

ASK YOUR DOCTOR

ELECTRO-CARDIOGRAPHY

Q Is it possible to get an electric shock when you have electrocardiography?

A There is absolutely no danger when you have an ECG. In this test, electricity that originates in your heart flows from you to the ECG machine. No electricity passes into you from the machine.

Q I recently had an ECG that turned out to be normal. My doctor now wants me to have an "exercise" ECG. What is this?

A Some heart disorders become evident only on an ECG done during exercise. If the arteries to your heart are narrowed as a result of coronary heart disease, the resting ECG may be normal. However, a recording made during exertion, when the heart requires a larger blood supply, may reveal a problem. An exercise ECG is recorded while you walk on a treadmill or ride on a stationary bicycle. The test is stopped if any symptoms develop.

Q My grandfather fainted recently. Why did his doctor send him home wearing a device called a Holter monitor?

A One of the causes of fainting, especially in the elderly, is an abrupt change in the heart rate or rhythm. The Holter monitor will record every beat of your grand-father's heart for 24 hours or longer. Sometimes clues to the suspected altered heart rhythm can be obtained by reviewing the pattern of the heartbeat over an extended period.

IMAGING THE HEART AND BLOOD VESSELS

DOCTORS RELY ON images of the heart and circulatory system to help them investigate a wide range of disorders. Imaging the heart can reveal its shape and size, the pumping action of the heart muscle, the flow of blood in and out of the heart chambers, and the size, shape, and efficiency of the heart valves. Images of the blood vessels can reveal structural abnormalities and can help your doctor identify any obstruction to the flow of blood.

Imaging techniques used for looking at the heart and the blood vessels include simple X-ray techniques and those in which a contrast agent (a substance opaque to X-rays) is injected into the bloodstream. In radionuclide scanning, a radioactive substance is injected into the blood; as it passes through the heart, it gives information about its structure and function. Noninvasive techniques that are increasingly being used include ultrasound scanning and magnetic resonance imaging (MRI).

LOOKING AT THE HEART

Doctors image the heart to assess its function, to look for structural abnormalities, or to confirm a diagnosis.

Chest X-ray

A chest X-ray is a simple method of obtaining an image of the heart. In conjunction with an ECG (see page 50), it is usually the first diagnostic test your doctor uses. Having a chest X-ray is a quick

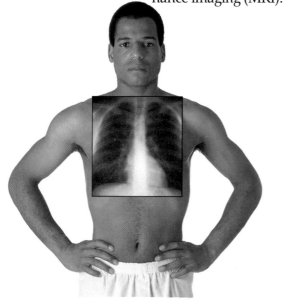

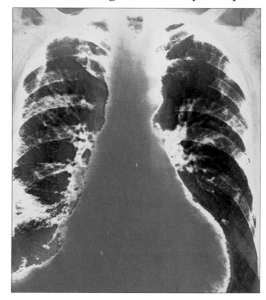

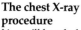

The chest X-ray procedure
You will be asked to stand and take a deep breath and hold it while two pictures are taken.

Chest X-ray views
The first picture is taken from the back with your hands on your hips and your elbows swung forward. This moves your shoulder blades outward so they do not obscure your lungs. The second view is taken from your right side with your arms held above your head.

Enlarged heart
This color-enhanced chest X-ray shows enlargement of the left ventricle in a person with high blood pressure. Enlargement of this part of the heart muscle is common in people with hypertension. The enlarged heart chamber is visible at the bottom right of the picture.

and painless procedure that is usually done on an outpatient basis.

A chest X-ray reveals the size, shape, and position of the heart and the large blood vessels that carry blood in and out of the heart chambers. Disorders that can be detected include enlargement of the heart chambers, ballooning of the upper part of the aorta, and expansion of the heart outline from accumulation of fluid in the pericardial sac.

A chest X-ray can confirm that the heart is failing to keep up with its work load by revealing accumulation of blood in the vessels, the presence of fluid inside the lungs, or an enlarged heart. Compared with some of the sophisticated imaging methods used today, the information gained from a chest X-ray is considered one-dimensional.

Coronary angiography

In this X-ray procedure, contrast medium is introduced into the coronary arteries, which supply the heart. X-rays are then taken so that the flow of blood through the arteries can be studied.

Coronary angiography is performed to reveal narrowing or blockage due to atherosclerosis. It helps the doctor decide whether the patient would benefit from treatment to widen or bypass the arteries (see BALLOON ANGIOPLASTY on page 118 and CORONARY ARTERY BYPASS on page 78). The technique for introducing the contrast medium is described later in this chapter (see CARDIAC CATHETERIZATION on page 60).

Echocardiography

Echocardiography is a widely used, harmless test that uses high-frequency sound waves (ultrasound) to produce a detailed picture of the heart. An instrument called a transducer, which produces a beam of sound waves, is held against your chest and directed toward different parts of your heart. The pattern of echoes is amplified by the transducer and displayed on a screen.

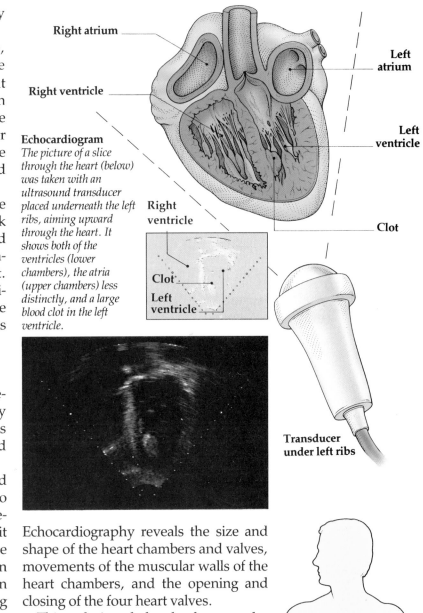

Echocardiogram
The picture of a slice through the heart (below) was taken with an ultrasound transducer placed underneath the left ribs, aiming upward through the heart. It shows both of the ventricles (lower chambers), the atria (upper chambers) less distinctly, and a large blood clot in the left ventricle.

Transducer under left ribs

Echocardiography reveals the size and shape of the heart chambers and valves, movements of the muscular walls of the heart chambers, and the opening and closing of the four heart valves.

This technique helps the doctor evaluate congenital heart defects in babies and adults. It also can detect a buildup of fluid around the heart, abnormal swelling of the chamber walls, or the presence of a blood clot in the heart chambers.

If a physical examination has revealed that you have a heart murmur, the doctor may refer you for echocardiography to find out if there is a damaged valve or if there is an abnormal communication between the chambers of your heart. Echocardiography is often performed after a heart attack to assess how well the damaged wall of the heart is contracting.

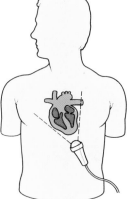

Transducer under ribs, aimed upward

Radionuclide scanning

In this procedure, a radioactive substance is injected into the bloodstream and carried around the circulation to the heart. Radiation that is detectable within the heart is then measured by a gamma camera, which contains a special crystal that reacts to rays of radiation (gamma rays) by emitting minute quantities of light (photons). The camera uses the photons to construct an image that is displayed on a monitor.

Radionuclide scanning provides useful information on how efficiently the heart is working but shows little anatomical detail. There are three types of radionuclide scanning used to image the heart – thallium scanning, technetium scanning, and cardiac blood pool imaging. The principles are similar, but slightly different information is obtained.

Does radionuclide scanning hurt?
This procedure is painless, except for the momentary pinprick sensation felt when the radioactive substance is injected.

Gamma camera

Is it safe?
Only tiny amounts of radiation are used, so radionuclide scanning is safe and there is a limited risk of toxic or allergic reactions.

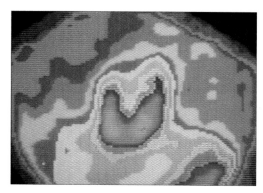

Thallium scan
This radionuclide scan of a normal heart was taken after injecting radioactive thallium into the bloodstream. The thallium has been taken up by healthy heart muscle (the red, horseshoe-shaped area). There are no cold spots. If there were, they would indicate areas not receiving sufficient oxygen.

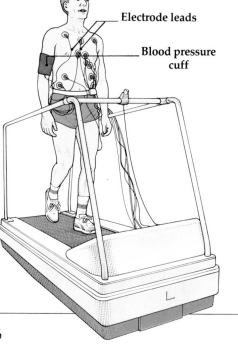

Electrode leads

Blood pressure cuff

Thallium scanning

Radioactive thallium is injected into a vein. It travels to the heart, where it is absorbed by healthy muscle but not by damaged muscle or areas that have a poor blood supply. Any area that has not absorbed thallium shows up as a "cold spot" on the scan. Heart muscle that has been partially destroyed by a heart attack appears as a persistent cold spot. A single thallium scan cannot distinguish between old and recent muscle damage.

If you have had symptoms such as chest pain or severe breathlessness brought on by exertion, you may have an exercise stress test that employs thallium. This type of thallium scan may also be performed to assess the effectiveness of coronary artery bypass surgery.

Thallium scanning takes between 45 and 90 minutes. You will be asked to return in 2 to 4 hours for another scan if the results of the first are positive. This helps the doctor differentiate damaged heart muscle from dead heart muscle. You should not use any alcohol, tobacco, or nonprescribed drugs for 24 hours before an exercise thallium scan.

Exercise thallium scanning
Throughout the period that you are walking on a treadmill, your pulse and blood pressure will be monitored and an ECG will be used to display the electrical activity in your heart. Shortly before the end of the test you will be given an injection of thallium. When the test is finished, you will be asked to lie under the scanner. If your blood pressure begins to fall during exercise, if the ECG shows any abnormal changes, or if adverse symptoms develop, you will be helped off the treadmill.

Technetium scanning

In this procedure, radioactive technetium pyrophosphate is injected into a vein. This substance is absorbed into areas of recently damaged heart muscle, but is not taken up by healthy muscle. Muscle partially destroyed by a heart attack appears as a "hot spot."

Technetium scanning is used to confirm a recent heart attack if ECG and blood tests have been inconclusive. It may also be used to determine the extent of the damage. Hot spots appear within 12 hours of a heart attack and usually disappear after a week.

A technetium scan takes between 30 and 60 minutes. The injection, which is given between 2 and 3 hours before the scan, occasionally causes mild discomfort, which wears off within minutes.

Cardiac blood pool imaging

Another radioactive technetium compound can be tagged onto red blood cells or albumin (a blood protein) and injected into a vein. A gamma camera is then positioned over the chest to provide images of the tagged blood as it flows in and out of the heart. The change in radioactivity each time the heart beats shows the doctor how much and how efficiently the heart is pumping.

The gamma camera can be set up to record the radiation at specific stages of the pumping cycle. In a multiple-gated acquisition (MUGA) scan, the camera records the emission of gamma rays at between 14 and 64 specific points during each heartbeat. The images produced are similar to the frames of a film and can be used to evaluate the movements of the heart muscle wall and changes in the volume of blood within each heart chamber. This allows the doctor to determine how well the heart is ejecting blood, which helps him or her establish the efficiency of the heartbeat. The MUGA scan may also be done while you are exercising to see how efficiently your heart responds to the extra work load.

Cardiac blood pool imaging
These two images, taken by the radioactive scanning technique called cardiac blood pool imaging, show the difference in blood distribution in the heart between diastole (when the heart is filling with blood) and systole (when the heart contracts). The color-coding represents gamma radiation from red blood cells labeled with a technetium-based radioactive tracer.

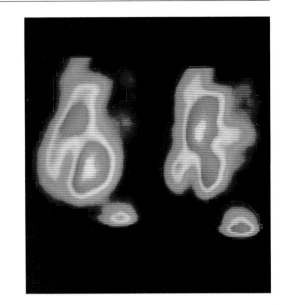

Positron emission tomography (PET) scanning

In PET scanning, a substance that takes part in biochemical processes in the body, such as carbon, nitrogen, or oxygen, is radioactively tagged and then injected into a vein. The substance travels to the heart, where it is taken up in greater concentrations by muscle cells that are more metabolically active. Positrons (positively charged particles) emitted by the radioactive substance cause the release of minute quantities of energy in the form of gamma rays. A ring of detectors positioned around your chest records the point of origin of the gamma rays and constructs a two- or three-dimensional image that reflects the level of metabolic activity in different parts of the heart muscle.

PET scanning is useful in pinpointing areas of the heart where activity is reduced or absent. Causes include impaired blood flow through heart muscle that has been damaged or destroyed as a result of long-standing coronary heart disease or immediately following a heart attack. The technique is particularly valuable in predicting whether the heart will recover after a heart attack or whether it will benefit from a coronary artery bypass, which is performed to reestablish an adequate flow of blood.

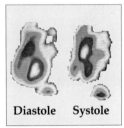

Diastole   Systole

SINGLE PHOTON EMISSION COMPUTED TOMOGRAPHY (SPECT)

SPECT is a specialized type of radionuclide scan. After injection of a radioactive substance, the gamma camera, which detects the radiation emitted, is rotated around your chest. A computer constructs cross-sectional images of your heart from the readings. This scan provides a more detailed picture of the damage to and circulation through heart structures than an ordinary radionuclide scan.

Rapid computed tomography (CT) scanning

CT scanning is a technique in which images of body slices are constructed using a computer and X-ray beams that are passed through the body at different angles. Until recently, CT scanning of the heart was unsatisfactory because the movement of the heart muscle produced a blurred picture. The development of a new type of CT scanner, which operates extremely rapidly, enables doctors to take pictures of the heart muscle in which the movement is frozen at different stages of the pumping cycle.

Magnetic resonance imaging (MRI)

MRI is a new technique that produces a high-quality image of the heart and major blood vessels, and of blood flow through the different chambers. The procedure reveals changes in the thickness of the heart muscle caused by damage from a heart attack. It can also be used to evaluate a congenital heart defect and to test how well a graft is working after coronary artery bypass surgery.

For MRI, you lie inside a large magnet that causes some of the atomic nuclei in your body to line up in parallel lines. Brief pulses of radio waves are passed

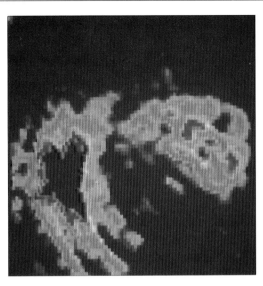

PET scan
This scan shows a slice through the heart. The light portions correspond to areas of the heart muscle that are receiving a good supply of oxygen.

3-D MRI scan
The three-dimensional image of the heart shown below was constructed by a computer from data obtained by magnetic resonance imaging. The image shows the top surface of the heart and the large blood vessels emerging from it.

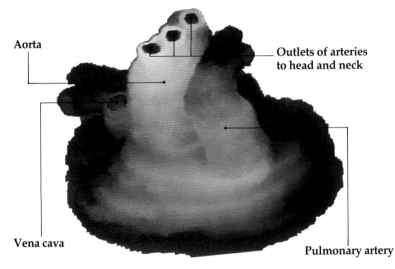

Aorta

Outlets of arteries to head and neck

Vena cava

Pulmonary artery

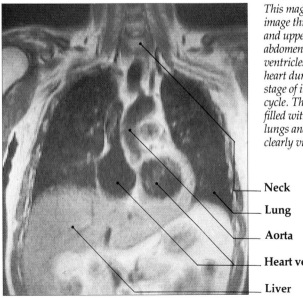

MRI chest scan
This magnetic resonance image through the chest and upper part of the abdomen shows the ventricles of a normal heart during the relaxed stage of its pumping cycle. The ventricles are filled with blood. The lungs and liver are also clearly visible.

Neck

Lung

Aorta

Heart ventricles

Liver

through your chest, knocking the atomic nuclei in their path out of line. Between pulses, the nuclei move back into line under the influence of the magnetic field and, as they do, release a radio signal. Different tissues emit signals of different strengths and frequencies. Areas that show hemorrhage, scarring, fluid overload, or insufficient blood supply have differing concentrations of the hydrogen atom and, thus, emit different radiofrequency signals. The MRI machine detects the radio signals and a computer produces an image from them.

MRI is painless and uses no radiation. It is not used on patients who have pacemakers because the magnetic field causes the pacemaker to malfunction.

LOOKING AT THE BLOOD VESSELS

Doctors image the arteries and veins to search for congenital abnormalities and to detect obstruction of normal blood flow, which may be due to deposits of fat in vessel walls, to blood clots, or to inflammation of the artery wall.

Angiography

Angiography is an X-ray procedure that reveals the outline of one or several arteries. First, a contrast medium is injected through a catheter into the artery being examined. The doctor then takes a series of X-ray pictures so that the flow of the contrast medium through the artery can be studied in detail.

Angiography can reveal narrowing or blockage of an artery, abnormal ballooning of an artery, bleeding from a damaged artery, or a change in the pattern of the vessels caused by a tumor.

This procedure is often given a specific name to describe the region being examined. For example, carotid angiography is used to look at the carotid arteries in the neck that supply blood to the brain.

Venography

In venography, contrast medium is injected into the vein under examination and a series of X-ray pictures is taken so that flow through the vein can be reviewed in detail.

Venography demonstrates abnormal narrowing or blockage of a vein caused by a blood clot or compression from a surrounding tumor. It is often performed to determine whether obstruction of a vein is the cause of a swollen arm or leg. Venography can also detect congenital abnormalities of veins and bleeding from damaged vessels. The veins most frequently examined are those in the leg, which is a common site for blood clots that tend to break off and flow to the pulmonary artery.

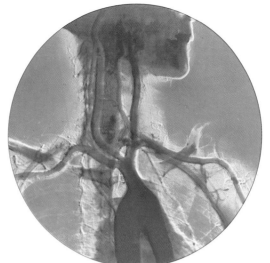

Color-enhanced angiogram
The image at left shows the arteries in the neck, shoulders, and upper part of the chest of a healthy person.

DIGITAL SUBTRACTION ANGIOGRAPHY

This relatively new type of angiography uses a computer to remove unwanted background information, so the image of the arteries stands out more clearly.

Venogram
This image of the upper part of the arm, taken after injection of a contrast medium, shows a vein, just above the elbow, blocked by a blood clot (arrow). No blood flow is visible above the clot. Also visible are another major vein, the bone, and several minor veins.

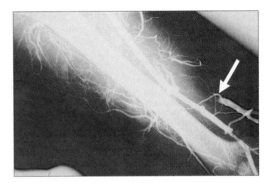

HOW DOPPLER ULTRASOUND WORKS

The doctor directs a beam of ultrasound waves at a blood vessel from a hand-held transducer. The echoes that are returned from the moving blood cells are recorded. They are then used to measure the speed and volume of blood flowing through the vessel.

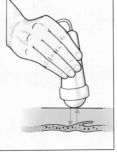

Doppler ultrasound

Doppler ultrasound works on the principle that, if the source of a sound is moving, the pitch (frequency) of the note will change. If the source of a sound gets closer, the note gets higher; if the source is moving away, the note gets lower. Called the Doppler effect, it is demonstrated by the changing note heard on a police siren as it moves past you.

The Doppler effect is used to study the flow of blood through vessels by aiming ultrasound waves at the vessels and then recording the changes in frequency of the echoes that are reflected. Doppler ultrasound is safe and painless and can be done in less than 20 minutes.

Color-flow Doppler ultrasound is a new technique in which the blood within the arteries and veins appears in color on the ultrasound monitor, with the color dependent upon the speed and uniformity of blood flow.

CARDIAC CATHETERIZATION

CARDIAC CATHETERIZATION consists of passing a soft tube, known as a catheter, through a vein or artery into the heart. This procedure may sound frightening, but it involves few risks, little discomfort, and can be of great value in diagnosis. Without it, many of the major advances in heart surgery that have been made in recent years would have been impossible.

Catheterization of the right side of the heart
This color-enhanced X-ray of the chest shows the catheter as a delicate curved line in the heart. Once in position, the catheter can be used to measure blood pressure inside the heart, to withdraw blood to measure blood gases, or, as shown here, to inject dye into the cavities or main blood vessels emerging from the heart so that X-ray photographs can be taken.

Cardiac catheterization is used most often to investigate coronary heart disease. However, it is also invaluable in the study of heart valve disease, heart defects in newborns and older children, and various other heart disorders. It can often provide a positive diagnosis when the results of other tests have been inconclusive. The technique is performed on people of all ages, from newborn babies to the elderly. In young children, the use of anesthesia is necessary. However, in older children, adolescents, and adults, the procedure is usually done under simple sedation.

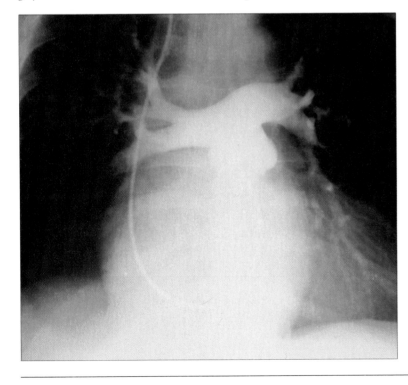

THE USES OF CATHETERIZATION

Catheterization enables doctors to obtain vital information about the structure and efficiency of the heart and circulatory system. It allows sampling of blood from the different chambers of the heart so that the gases can be analyzed and information obtained about possible defects in the structure of the heart and the functioning of the circulatory system. It also allows blood pressure readings to be made at different points in the heart. For example, the state of the heart valves can be investigated by comparing the blood pressure on either side of the valves. Such readings can help evaluate the extent of a valve defect and assess the heart's pumping efficiency.

During the procedure, fluids opaque to X-rays may be injected into the heart chambers, or injected directly into the coronary arteries (see CORONARY ANGIOGRAPHY on page 55). Injecting dye allows the chambers of the heart to be seen on a monitor and allows a videotape recording to be made.

In addition to its function in diagnosis, cardiac catheterization has become an important and growing aid to treatment. Balloon catheters are being used to open up narrowed coronary arteries and to dilate tightly narrowed heart valves (see BALLOON ANGIOPLASTY on page 118).

CATHETERIZATION OF THE RIGHT AND LEFT SIDES OF THE HEART

Different routes of catheterization are used according to whether measurements are to be made (or treatment performed) in the right or left sides of the heart.

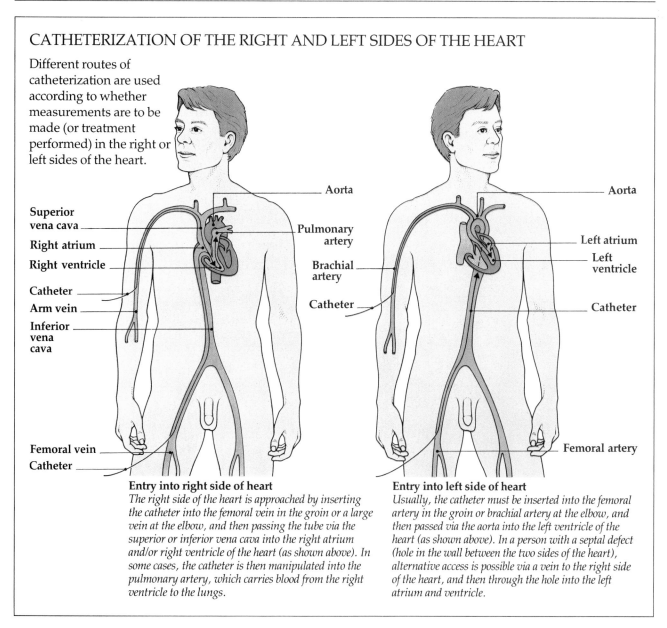

Aorta

Superior vena cava

Right atrium

Right ventricle

Catheter

Arm vein

Inferior vena cava

Pulmonary artery

Aorta

Left atrium

Left ventricle

Brachial artery

Catheter

Catheter

Femoral vein

Catheter

Femoral artery

Entry into right side of heart
The right side of the heart is approached by inserting the catheter into the femoral vein in the groin or a large vein at the elbow, and then passing the tube via the superior or inferior vena cava into the right atrium and/or right ventricle of the heart (as shown above). In some cases, the catheter is then manipulated into the pulmonary artery, which carries blood from the right ventricle to the lungs.

Entry into left side of heart
Usually, the catheter must be inserted into the femoral artery in the groin or brachial artery at the elbow, and then passed via the aorta into the left ventricle of the heart (as shown above). In a person with a septal defect (hole in the wall between the two sides of the heart), alternative access is possible via a vein to the right side of the heart, and then through the hole into the left atrium and ventricle.

PERFORMING CARDIAC CATHETERIZATION

The procedure involves the insertion of a long, fine, flexible tube, made of a material opaque to X-rays, into a vein or artery. The tube is carefully manipulated along the vessel, under X-ray control, until the tip reaches the desired point, either inside the heart or in an artery. During catheterization, the state of the heart's action is monitored continuously by an electrocardiograph. If you are having cardiac catheterization, you are asked to lie fairly still, in different positions, for up to 45 minutes. The entire test may last from 2 to 3 hours.

What does it feel like?
Catheterization usually causes only slight discomfort; the presence of the catheter in the heart causes no sensation. Coronary angiography can be slightly uncomfortable. During the injection of the contrast medium, patients may experience a flushing, warm or hot sensation all over the body, a metallic taste in the mouth, or nausea. These sensations usually last for only a few minutes.

WHAT ARE THE RISKS?

Cardiac catheterization does not usually cause any complications, though some people experience an allergic reaction to the contrast medium that is injected. In rarer cases, there is damage to the artery into which the catheter is inserted.

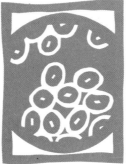

BLOOD AND FLUID TESTS

LABORATORY ANALYSIS of blood and body fluids supplies valuable information about the condition of the heart. For example, measuring certain enzyme levels in the blood after a heart attack gives the doctor an indication of the severity of heart muscle damage. Estimating the level of cholesterol in a person's blood helps identify one of the risks of heart disease.

BLOOD LIPID LEVELS

Research studies in hospital laboratories and on populations have proven that there is a distinct link between the risk of a heart attack and the amount of cholesterol in your blood. The risk is especially high if your cholesterol consistently exceeds 240 milligrams per 100 milliliters of blood. Raised levels tend to run in some families. If anyone in your family has had a heart attack before age 50, you should have your cholesterol tested. All adults 20 years and older should have their cholesterol level measured at least once. Blood lipid tests can be misleading if they are done within 3 months after a heart attack. Even a minor illness can cause a reduction in blood cholesterol, so figures taken at that time are not reliable.

An enzyme is a protein that regulates the rate of a chemical reaction in the body. Whenever any body tissue is injured, certain enzymes within the cells are released into the bloodstream. This process occurs when blockage of a coronary artery injures, and sometimes kills, part of the heart muscle. Measuring the enzyme levels in the blood reflects how much of the heart muscle has been damaged by a heart attack.

MEASURING HEART ENZYME LEVELS

The amount of enzymes varies in different tissues, so, if several enzyme measurements are taken, it is sometimes possible to confirm that the heart has been damaged and not a muscle elsewhere in the body. The enzymes are present in the body cells in much higher concentrations than they are in the blood, so even minor tissue damage can cause a rise in the enzyme levels in the blood. Many different enzymes are released from heart tissue after a heart attack, but only some of them are selected for measurement. These enzymes are chosen because they are easiest to measure and are detectable in very small amounts.

How are enzyme levels measured?

Enzymes are, by their nature, highly active chemical substances; it is usually

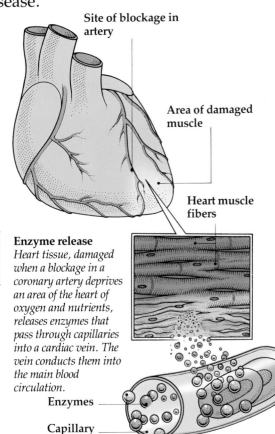

Site of blockage in artery

Area of damaged muscle

Heart muscle fibers

Enzyme release
Heart tissue, damaged when a blockage in a coronary artery deprives an area of the heart of oxygen and nutrients, releases enzymes that pass through capillaries into a cardiac vein. The vein conducts them into the main blood circulation.

Enzymes

Capillary

easier to measure their activity than their concentration. For this reason, blood enzyme estimations are usually expressed in international units of enzyme activity.

The heart enzyme levels most commonly estimated are aspartate aminotransferase, lactate dehydrogenases, and creatine kinase. A subset of the latter, MB fraction creatine kinase (CK-MB) isoenzyme, is especially useful because heart muscle is the only tissue in the body containing more than 5 percent

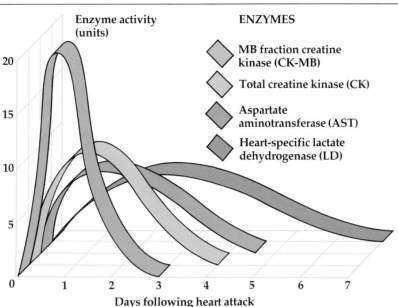

Enzyme activity
After a heart attack there is no change in enzyme activity for several hours. Enzyme activity then rises rapidly to a peak, subsiding over the following few days at a rate that varies according to the type of enzyme. The graph charts the "behavior" of four selected enzymes over the course of 1 week. By the end of the week, enzyme activity has returned to its original level.

ENZYMES

◆ MB fraction creatine kinase (CK-MB)

◆ Total creatine kinase (CK)

◆ Aspartate aminotransferase (AST)

◆ Heart-specific lactate dehydrogenase (LD)

BACTERIAL ENDOCARDITIS

Bacterial endocarditis, an infection of the heart valve linings, is a life-threatening condition that can destroy the heart valves. The early symptoms are loss of energy, appetite, and weight. There may be fever and chills, anemia, clubbing of the fingers, and tiny hemorrhages, which look like slivers, under the nails. The streptococci responsible (below) circulate in the bloodstream.

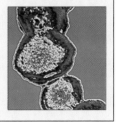

CK-MB. One of the lactate dehydrogenase levels is also very useful because its activity in the blood remains raised for a much longer period than the activity of the other enzymes.

For maximum information, blood samples are taken within 18 to 30 hours after the start of a heart attack. Later measurements of enzyme activity usually show a return to normal levels, indicating no further damage to the heart tissue. A combination of electrocardiogram and enzyme estimation can confirm or refute a diagnosis of myocardial infarction (heart attack) with almost 100 percent certainty.

ROUTINE BLOOD ANALYSIS

Any heart disorder is made worse if you are anemic. Doctors check for anemia with a blood test. The complete blood cell count and the erythrocyte sedimentation rate (the rate at which red blood cells settle in a standing blood sample) may be important in the diagnosis of infectious and inflammatory heart conditions. Changes in the serum electrolyte levels (electrically charged substances in the blood) are sometimes important. When these levels are abnormal, they may severely affect the electrical conducting system of the heart.

Hormone levels

The level of hormones produced by the endocrine glands may also be important. The heart is affected by overactivity of the thyroid gland, and overproduction of steroid hormones by the adrenal glands can raise the blood pressure. An increased output of epinephrine and norepinephrine from a tumor of the adrenal glands can also affect the heart.

PERICARDIAL FLUID ASPIRATION

Fluid sometimes collects between the heart and the sac (called the pericardium) that surrounds it, interfering with the heart's action. Using an ultrasound transducer to guide the needle, the doctor removes the fluid and sends it to the laboratory for examination and culture. The presence of fluid suggests that the pericardium is inflamed, which may be caused by an immune disorder, viruses, or tubercle bacilli. Fluid may also accumulate as a result of hormonal and biochemical disorders, as well as some malignant growths.

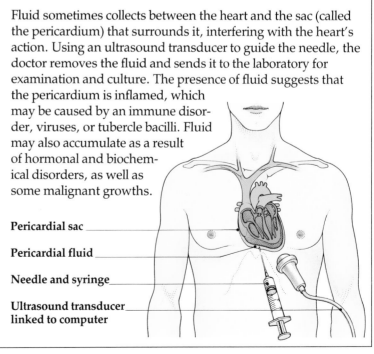

Pericardial sac

Pericardial fluid

Needle and syringe

Ultrasound transducer linked to computer

CHAPTER FIVE

DISORDERS OF THE HEART

DESPITE THE OVERALL reduction in the incidence of heart disease over the last 25 years, about half of all Americans will have a problem affecting their heart or circulation at some time in their lives. At any time about one quarter of the population is affected. This chapter reviews the causes, symptoms, and treatment of the most common heart disorders. By far the most important disorder affecting the heart is coronary heart disease – the underlying cause of angina, myocardial infarctions (heart attacks), and most heart rhythm disturbances (arrhythmias). Coronary heart disease affects an estimated 6 million Americans and causes about 1,500 deaths every day in the US. In the following pages, you will learn how it develops, the symptoms it causes, and the exact way in which it damages the heart. Also included are special features on living with angina and on life after a heart attack, with the emphasis on life-style changes to reduce your chances of a second attack. Other important disorders covered include congenital heart disease, which affects an estimated 25,000 infants born each year in the US; heart valve disorders, which afflict up to 2 million Americans; heart failure, which disables more than 2 million citizens; and

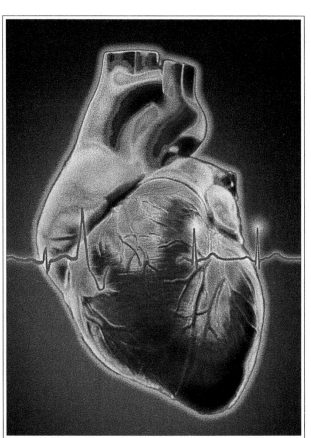

the various types of heart muscle disease (cardiomyopathy). High blood pressure (hypertension) – the most common of all disorders affecting the cardiovascular system – is examined in detail in Chapter Six. Several of the more important symptom patterns of heart disorders – and the way they are diagnosed and treated – are illustrated in this chapter by CASE HISTORY features. The MONITOR YOUR SYMPTOMS charts and the section on SYMPTOMS OF HEART AND CIRCULATORY DISEASE will guide you to the possible causes of symptoms such as chest pain, palpitations, and swollen ankles. The ASK YOUR DOCTOR columns will answer your questions on topics ranging from holes in the heart to irregular heart rhythms.

More than 2 million operations on the cardiovascular system are performed annually in US hospitals. The SURGICAL PROCEDURES boxes illustrate several important surgical treatments for heart disorders, including heart valve replacement, the correction of a congenital heart defect, coronary artery bypass surgery, and heart transplant operations. In recent years, the continually improving success rates from such operations, together with improvements in drug treatment, have played a significant part in the lowering of death rates from heart problems in the US.

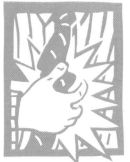

SYMPTOMS OF HEART AND CIRCULATORY DISEASE

HEART AND CIRCULATORY DISORDERS may make themselves apparent by causing a wide variety of symptoms, such as breathlessness during exertion or at rest, swollen ankles, chest pain, palpitations, dizziness, and fainting. However, many other health problems – some of them trivial – also cause these symptoms. If you have experienced any of these symptoms, it does not necessarily indicate that there is something wrong with your heart.

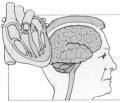

DIZZINESS
Most attacks of dizziness, in which you feel unsteady and lightheaded for a few seconds, are harmless. Recurrent attacks of dizziness may be due to a heart or circulatory problem. One uncommon cause is heart block (see page 98). An impaired flow of blood to the brain may cause a transient ischemic attack (see page 121).

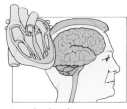

FAINTING
A fainting attack is a temporary loss of consciousness due to a lack of oxygen reaching the brain. Fainting is usually harmless and is frequently the result of standing for a long time in a hot or stuffy atmosphere. Sometimes it is caused by overstimulation of the vagus nerve (which helps control the heart rate) brought on by severe pain or a sudden shock. In rare cases, fainting is the result of heart block or a transient ischemic attack. Anyone who faints during exercise should have the cause investigated immediately; it can be a symptom of a serious heart disorder.

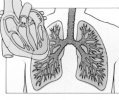

BREATHLESSNESS
People usually become out of breath when they exercise strenuously because the lungs must work harder to keep the heart and other muscles supplied with oxygen. This is normal. However, if you are breathless when you are resting or doing some nonstrenuous exercise it may be a symptom of a heart problem.

A common cause of breathlessness, especially in the elderly, is heart failure (see page 104). The heart pumps the blood less efficiently, slowing the flow of blood through the lungs. This results in breathlessness, partly because the lungs cannot maintain an adequate supply of oxygen to the circulation, and partly because the reduced output of the heart allows fluid to accumulate in the lung tissues.

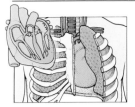

CHEST PAIN

Chest pain is extremely common and is often caused by a strained muscle, a broken rib, a trapped nerve, psychological stress, irritation of the esophagus, or inflammation of a rib joint to one side of the breastbone. In some people, the pain is caused by a heart disorder such as angina (see page 74), a heart attack (see page 78), or pericarditis (see page 94).

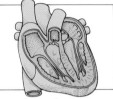

PALPITATIONS

Palpitations are fluttering or thumping sensations in the chest or neck that make you aware of your own heartbeat. Some people suffer palpitations when they are tense, others when they feel calm and rested. Palpitations can be caused by an ectopic heartbeat (an isolated, irregular beat), which can be frightening but is not usually due to any heart disorder.

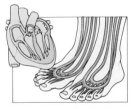

SWOLLEN ANKLES

Swelling of the ankles is a symptom of fluid retention in the tissues. One of several causes is heart failure (see page 104), in which the heart's ventricles do not empty properly. Blood retained in the right ventricle causes a buildup of blood and consequent pressure through the circulation, forcing fluid out into the surrounding tissues. The ankles, in particular, become swollen because the effect of gravity pulls the fluid down.

TREATING HEART FAILURE

Symptoms that arise as a result of heart failure, such as some cases of breathlessness or swollen ankles, occur because the poor functioning of the heart causes fluid to be forced out of the circulation and into the surrounding tissues. It is important to reduce the accumulation of fluid. For this reason, the symptoms are treated with diuretic drugs. The drugs act by interfering with the functioning of the kidneys, reducing the amount of salt and water that is reabsorbed from them into the bloodstream. Thus more fluid is expelled in the urine. The drug digitalis helps heart failure by improving the contractile strength of the heart muscle.

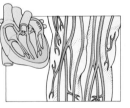

CRAMP

This muscle spasm usually results from strenuous exercise. If it occurs after walking a short distance and stops with rest, it is called intermittent claudication (see page 122) and indicates arterial diseases.

ASK YOUR DOCTOR

CIRCULATORY DISORDERS

Q I suffer from cold hands and feet. Does this mean that I have a circulation problem?

A Cold hands and feet are not necessarily a symptom of blocked or narrowed blood vessels in the limbs. Your doctor can reassure you by examining your circulation, checking your pulse, and looking at the color of your skin. However, cold hands and feet associated with pain, pallor, or discoloration may be a sign of a circulatory disorder or may occur as a side effect of drugs such as beta blockers.

Q I have been having headaches and nosebleeds. Could they be due to hypertension?

A Probably not. Causes such as a sinus infection and/or a very dry atmosphere in your home are more likely. Most people with high blood pressure (hypertension) feel fine until a complication (such as stroke, heart attack, or heart failure) develops.

Q Both of my ankles swell after I've been on my feet all day. Do you think I have a heart problem?

A The most common cause of ankle swelling is congestion of blood in your leg veins, not heart failure. Standing for long periods causes a buildup of blood in those veins, and the resulting back pressure forces fluid out of the circulation to cause edema (swelling). After your doctor has checked your heart and circulation, the best treatment for ankle swelling due to venous congestion is regular exercise and keeping your legs raised when you relax at the end of the day.

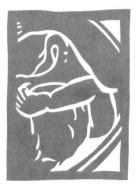

CONGENITAL HEART DISEASE

ABOUT ONE PERSON in 140 is born with a congenital heart defect. The term congenital means "present from birth," though some abnormalities are in fact detected before birth, and some not until childhood or even adolescence. Thanks to major advances in diagnosis and surgery over the last 30 years, most defects can now be successfully repaired. Some are so mild they require no treatment.

Congenital heart defects are anatomical abnormalities caused by the defective development of the heart during fetal life. They include such abnormalities as septal defects (holes in the heart), misplacements of major vessels, single ventricles, and numerous other disorders of varying severity. Septal defects form the largest and most common group of major birth defects.

There are many types of defects (the chart on page 69 shows some of the most common ones), but they can be divided into two basic types – those that cause too much blood to pass from the heart to the lungs, and not enough to the body, and those that cause insufficient blood to pass to the lungs, causing the blood that goes to the body to contain an insufficient amount of oxygen.

CAUSES

The heart forms in the early weeks of pregnancy, between the sixth and 12th week, which is often before a woman even realizes that she is pregnant. If a pregnant woman contracts a virus infection at this time, particularly rubella (German measles), there is a possibility that a heart abnormality will develop in her child. Routine rubella vaccination in childhood has made this infection during pregnancy extremely rare in the US today, but other viral infections may also affect a baby's heart.

Poorly controlled diabetes in a pregnant woman also seems to increase the risk of a heart defect in the child. Congenital heart disease often accompanies congenital abnormalities that affect other parts of the body. About 30 to 40 percent of babies born with Down's syndrome have a heart defect. There is also a slight increase in the incidence of some types of defects in twins.

Clubbing of fingers
Prolonged cyanosis, which is a bluish complexion caused by insufficient oxygen in the blood, can lead to thickening and broadening of the fingers and toes (clubbing), with an increase in the curvature of the nails. The lower photograph shows finger clubbing in a young child with a congenital heart defect. The upper photograph shows cyanosis and clubbing of the fingers in an older child with the complex of congenital heart defects called tetralogy of Fallot.

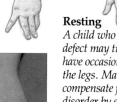

Resting
A child who has a heart defect may tire easily and have occasional cramps in the legs. Many children compensate for their disorder by squatting down spontaneously to take a rest.

CONGENITAL DEFECTS

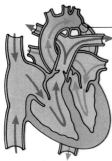

Region of aortic narrowing

Coarctation of the aorta

This is a tight, localized narrowing of the aorta, which reduces the supply of blood to the lower part of the body. It leads to breathlessness, pallor, and the inability to feed. Emergency surgery may be necessary in the second week of life, but sometimes surgery is delayed until the child is 4 to 6 years old.

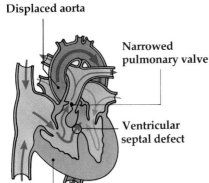

Displaced aorta

Narrowed pulmonary valve

Ventricular septal defect

Thickened wall

Tetralogy of Fallot

This is a combination of four anomalies – a narrowed valve in the pulmonary artery leading to the lungs, a hole in the partition between the two pumping parts of the heart (ventricular septal defect), a displaced aorta that overrides the partition, and an abnormally thickened wall of the right ventricle. Insufficient blood passes to the lungs to be oxygenated, and the large volume pumped to the body thus lacks oxygen, leading to breathlessness. Surgery is required.

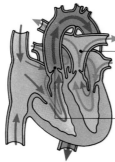

Pulmonary artery arises from the left ventricle

Aorta arises from the right ventricle

Transposition of the great vessels

In this defect, the two main arteries (the pulmonary artery and the aorta) that carry blood from the heart arise from the wrong sides of the heart. Surgery is performed to disconnect and then reposition the misplaced vessels.

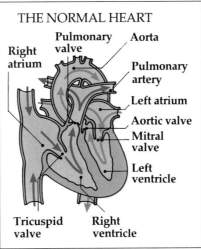

THE NORMAL HEART

Right atrium

Pulmonary valve

Aorta

Pulmonary artery

Left atrium

Aortic valve

Mitral valve

Left ventricle

Tricuspid valve

Right ventricle

Atrial septal defect

Atrial septal defect

This is a hole in the partition between the two atria, which results in too much blood flowing to the lungs. An operation may be performed at age 4 or 5.

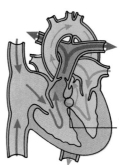

Ventricular septal defect

Ventricular septal defect

This is a hole in the partition between the main pumping chambers of the heart. Some of the red, oxygenated blood from the left ventricle passes through the hole to the right ventricle, which results in too much blood flowing to the lungs. This defect tends to shrink as the child grows; it often closes completely. Only large defects require surgery, which is usually performed before age 2, to patch the hole.

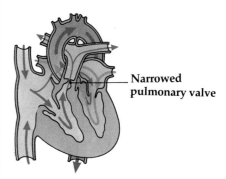

Narrowed pulmonary valve

Pulmonary stenosis

In this defect, there is a narrowing of the pulmonary valve, which forces the heart muscle to work harder to push the blood through the narrowed area. The degree of narrowing may be mild, moderate, or severe; surgery is required only in the most severe cases. Balloon dilatation has been used to widen the narrowing without the need for surgery in some children. There are rarely any symptoms. If surgery is not required, the child's condition is monitored every 2 to 3 years.

No known cause

In most cases, however, no cause can be found. If a child is born with a heart defect, it is certainly not the parents' fault. Feelings of guilt can greatly intensify what is already a very difficult situation for the parents.

Congenital is not synonymous with hereditary. It is rare, in fact, for more than one person to be affected in the same family. The risk of having a child with congenital heart disease if one parent has a heart abnormality, or if a couple has already had an affected child, is only slightly increased.

SYMPTOMS

The problems that are related to too much blood in the lungs and not enough in the body lead primarily to breathlessness and exhaustion; those leading to insufficient blood in the lungs and insufficient oxygen in the blood that goes to the body lead to blueness of the tissues, mainly of the lips and nails.

Before or at birth

Some abnormalities can be detected before birth when a pregnant woman has an ultrasound scan. Some are obvious immediately after birth, when a baby may become or remain blue, have labored breathing, or collapse suddenly, often while feeding. At this stage (immediately after birth), no definitive treat-

ment is usually required for less severe defects, which often resolve themselves naturally in the first year of life.

In babies that appear to be normal at birth, increasing breathlessness – leading to increasing difficulties in feeding – may appear after a few weeks.

Over 1 year old

Increasing blueness or breathlessness may become noticeable only after the end of the first year of life. In other cases, there may be no suspicion that any problem exists until abnormal turbulence results in a heart murmur, or abnormal circulation leads to irregularities in the child's pulse. These problems are sometimes first detected during a preschool or school medical examination.

Complications

A severe heart defect can be life-threatening at or soon after birth unless treated promptly. Some less severe defects can cause stunted growth and underdeveloped muscles and limbs. Repeated colds can lead to pneumonia. Prolonged cyanosis can lead to clubbing (widening of the tips) of the fingers and toes. A child may also tire rapidly and be unable to take part in physical exercise.

Respiratory distress
A congenital heart disorder that is producing too much blood in the lungs should be suspected if congestive heart failure occurs in early infancy. It may be indicated by breathlessness, feeding difficulties, and failure to thrive; the infant may have a weak cry and a tense, anxious face, with beads of perspiration on the forehead.

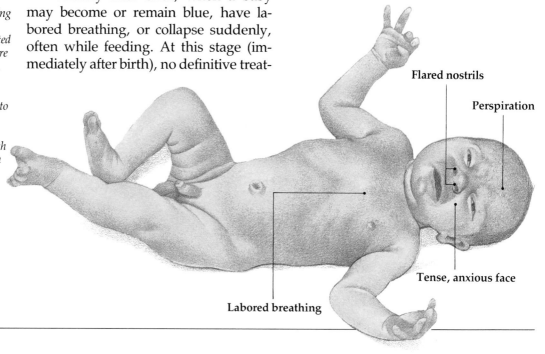

Flared nostrils

Perspiration

Tense, anxious face

Labored breathing

SURGICAL PROCEDURES
REPAIRING A HOLE IN THE HEART

A VENTRICULAR SEPTAL DEFECT – a hole between the heart's two pumping chambers – is a common congenital defect. A small hole seldom causes problems and often closes without treatment, but a large hole can be life-threatening. The doctor and parents must weigh the benefits of surgery against its risks. The most common operation is shown, though in a very young child a temporary palliative procedure may be performed first.

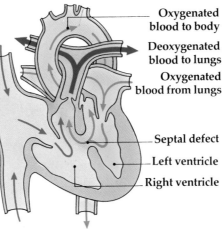

Oxygenated blood to body

Deoxygenated blood to lungs

Oxygenated blood from lungs

Septal defect

Left ventricle

Right ventricle

Ventricular septal defect
If there is a large hole between the two sides of the heart, much of the oxygenated blood returning to the left ventricle from the lungs is pumped through the hole to the right side of the heart and then to the lungs again. This causes overloading of the blood vessels in the lungs and an insufficient blood supply to the body.

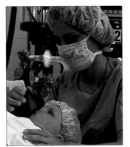

Site of incision

Septal defect

Plastic patch

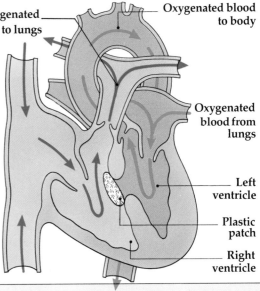

3 An incision is made in the thin wall of the right ventricle. A small, soft, plastic patch is used to close the septal defect. The patch is carefully and securely stitched into place, using tiny, curved, eyeless needles (right).

1 After a full preoperative examination, the patient is given a general anesthetic. On the operating table, the chest is opened by an incision in the breastbone. This allows the doctors access to the heart.

Stiches

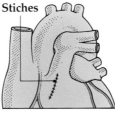

4 When the patch is in place, the wall of the ventricle is tightly closed with stitches that bring the edges of the muscle into close contact (left). The heart is then restarted and the heart-lung machine is disconnected.

Clamp

From heart-lung machine

Superior vena cava

Aorta

To heart-lung machine

Inferior vena cava

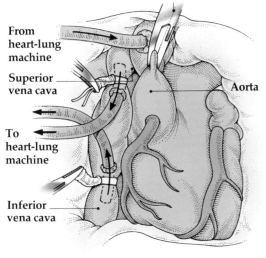

2 Venous blood returning to the right side of the heart is diverted to a heart-lung machine, where the blood is oxygenated and pumped back into the body. The heart is then completely stopped and emptied of blood.

Deoxygenated blood to lungs

Oxygenated blood to body

5 With the hole closed, the contractions of the left ventricle are able to pump blood to the body, while those of the right ventricle pump it to the lungs (right). There is no longer any mixing of the two circulations. The effects of surgery are dramatic, with a considerable improvement in the general condition of the patient.

Oxygenated blood from lungs

Left ventricle

Plastic patch

Right ventricle

ASK YOUR DOCTOR

CONGENITAL HEART DISEASE

Q My baby was born with a small hole in her heart. I'm told it will probably close. In the meantime, should she have all her inoculations?

A About a quarter of all holes in the heart close spontaneously. It's only when the hole is large that surgery may be required. Your baby should have all her routine inoculations. Only babies under 1 year who are acutely ill should have the inoculations postponed.

Q My first child was born with a congenital heart defect and needed an operation to correct it. She's fine now, but it was a frightening experience. I'd like to have another baby but am worried about a repeat performance. Is it likely?

A No. The risk is only slightly increased to about one in 50. It is comparatively rare for a woman to have two children who have a congenital heart defect.

Q Why is it important for children with congenital heart disease to be careful with their teeth?

A Children with heart defects are at risk of a serious infection known as endocarditis, which settles inside the heart. It can be caused by bacteria entering the blood via the mouth after dental treatment, so it is important to care for teeth from an early age by avoiding sweet foods and drinks, and brushing the teeth regularly using a fluoride toothpaste. Your dentist should be made aware of the situation and may, along with your doctor, recommend the use of antibiotics before any dental work.

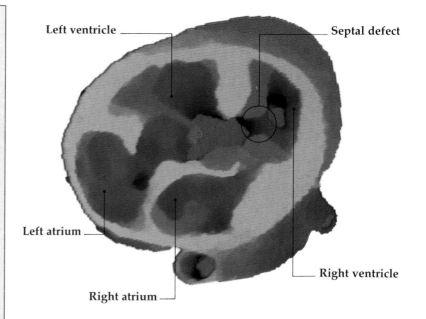

Left ventricle — Septal defect — Left atrium — Right ventricle — Right atrium —

DIAGNOSIS AND TREATMENT

Heart defects are often diagnosed before birth by ultrasound scanning. This technique is useful because it allows doctors to make preparations for emergency treatment at birth.

A heart defect may be suspected after a clinical examination and confirmed by several procedures, including X-rays, electrocardiography, echocardiography, and cardiac catheterization.

Treatment

Some conditions, such as small septal defects, may become less severe or disappear completely on their own. Rest, oxygen, and medication can be used to assist the circulation and lung function, sometimes improving the child's condition prior to surgery for a limited time or sometimes indefinitely.

Other defects are likely to worsen, in which case surgical correction may be the only answer. Some can be repaired with a single, relatively simple operation. Others require a temporary palliative treatment, followed by full corrective surgery later. In severe cases, a heart transplant may be a last resort.

Hole in the heart
A congenital septal defect, often referred to as a hole in the heart, may occur between the two upper chambers (atria) or the lower chambers (ventricles) of the heart. This 3-D magnetic resonance imaging (MRI) scan of a section through the heart shows a defect between the left and right ventricles.

AFTER SURGERY

Following successful heart surgery, recovery usually takes place rapidly, and most children have a normal, or at least near-normal, life expectancy. A full range of activities, including sports, is usually possible between 3 and 6 months after a successful operation.

CASE HISTORY
FATIGUE AND BREATHLESSNESS

JEREMY HAS APPEARED, up to now, to be a perfectly normal, healthy child. His mother became concerned when she noticed that Jeremy was having difficulty keeping up physically with his younger sister. In particular, although fond of games and swimming, Jeremy seemed to tire easily and was breathless after even the most minor effort.

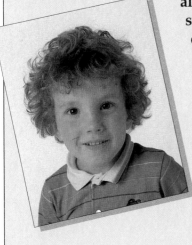

PERSONAL DETAILS
Name Jeremy Becker
Age 6
Occupation Schoolboy
Family Jeremy's family is in good health. He has a 4-year-old sister.

THE CONSULTATION

The doctor gives Jeremy a general physical examination and can't, at first, find anything wrong. Using her stethoscope, however, the doctor detects a fairly loud, continuous, rumbling sound between Jeremy's second and third ribs on the left side. This prompts her to suggest a consultation with a cardiologist.

THE SPECIALIST CONSULTATION

The cardiologist suggests that chest X-rays be taken. They show a slight enlargement of the heart and enlargement of the pulmonary arteries running from the heart to the lungs. The doctor uses echocardiography and Doppler ultrasound to confirm his suspicions.

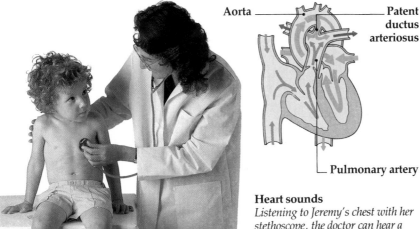

Aorta — Patent ductus arteriosus

Pulmonary artery

Heart sounds
Listening to Jeremy's chest with her stethoscope, the doctor can hear a continuous rumbling sound that prompts her to refer him to a cardiologist.

THE DIAGNOSIS

The cardiologist explains that, during fetal life, the lungs do not function. The blood, which after birth flows through the lungs, is shunted before birth through a short passage between the artery to the lungs (the pulmonary artery) and the main artery of the body (the aorta). This passage is called the ductus arteriosus. It normally closes after birth. If the duct remains open (patent), some of the blood pumped by the left side of the heart into the aorta is shunted through the duct into the circulation going to the lungs.

The open duct is called a PATENT DUCTUS ARTERIOSUS and all the findings, such as enlargement of the pulmonary arteries and the rumbling sound heard through the stethoscope, indicate that Jeremy is suffering from this defect. The result has been some retardation of his growth and development and an extra strain on his heart, which has caused breathlessness during exertion.

The specialist also explains that Jeremy is susceptible to a serious complication called endocarditis, which is an infection of the duct that may spread to the heart lining. He tells Jeremy's parents that Jeremy should have an immediate operation to close the abnormal pathway.

THE TREATMENT

Jeremy's operation is performed 2 weeks later, through a small incision in the side of his chest. The surgery consists of cutting through and tying off the ends of the ductus arteriosus. The operation takes an hour.

Within days of surgery, Jeremy is feeling well and energetic. Three months later, his heart is functioning normally. Within a year, his mother notices great progress in his physical development and his ability to keep up with his sister.

CORONARY HEART DISEASE

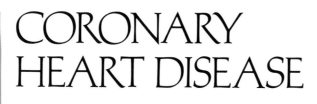

THE GENERAL TERM "coronary heart disease" describes a variety of different disorders of the heart muscle that are caused by restriction or blockage of its blood supply. The disorders range from the warning pain of angina to the injury and even death of parts of the heart muscle caused by a myocardial infarction, or heart attack.

Most coronary heart disease is the result of narrowing of the coronary arteries by atherosclerosis (see page 14).

ANGINA

Angina is pain – a symptom, not a disease. Angina pectoris simply means "pain in the chest." Angina occurs when the work demanded of your heart muscle exceeds the ability of the coronary arteries to supply the oxygen and fuel needed to perform it. Angina may be no more than a vague ache or difficulty breathing, but often it is a tight, gripping pain, sometimes of a crushing, frighten-

HOW BLOOD CIRCULATES THROUGH THE HEART

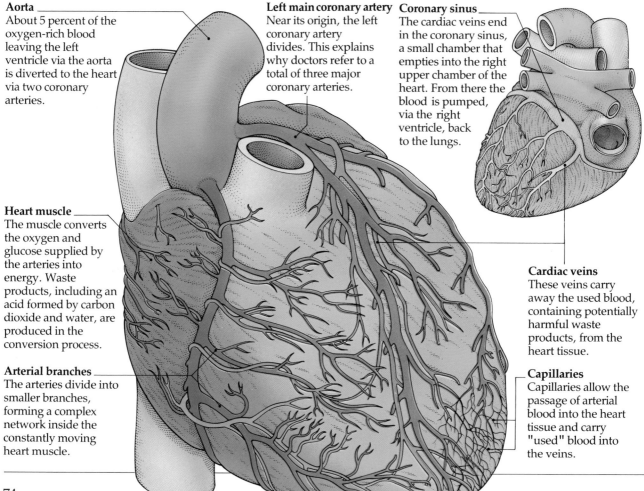

Aorta
About 5 percent of the oxygen-rich blood leaving the left ventricle via the aorta is diverted to the heart via two coronary arteries.

Left main coronary artery
Near its origin, the left coronary artery divides. This explains why doctors refer to a total of three major coronary arteries.

Coronary sinus
The cardiac veins end in the coronary sinus, a small chamber that empties into the right upper chamber of the heart. From there the blood is pumped, via the right ventricle, back to the lungs.

Heart muscle
The muscle converts the oxygen and glucose supplied by the arteries into energy. Waste products, including an acid formed by carbon dioxide and water, are produced in the conversion process.

Arterial branches
The arteries divide into smaller branches, forming a complex network inside the constantly moving heart muscle.

Cardiac veins
These veins carry away the used blood, containing potentially harmful waste products, from the heart tissue.

Capillaries
Capillaries allow the passage of arterial blood into the heart tissue and carry "used" blood into the veins.

WHAT CAUSES ANGINA?

Angina typically consists of a heavy, pressurelike discomfort behind the breastbone that is brought on by exercise – especially when the demand on the heart is increased by strong emotion or by a recent, heavy meal. Any pain that is brought on by effort and that spreads up into the neck, through to the back, or down the left arm, and disappears with rest, is almost certainly angina and should be fully investigated.

Contrary to popular belief, angina is seldom felt in the lower left part of the chest – the area in which the heartbeat is most easily felt. In unusual cases, angina does not occur in the chest at all, but only in the left arm, neck, or wrist.

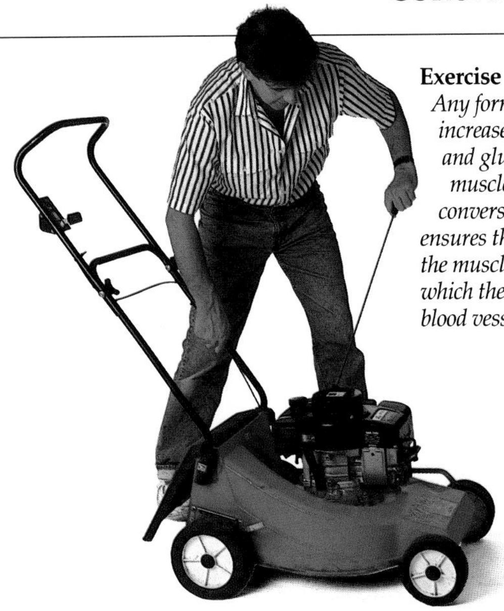

Exercise
Any form of strenuous exercise increases the body's need for oxygen and glucose, mainly because the muscles require them as fuel for conversion into energy. The body ensures that an adequate supply reaches the muscles by increasing the rate at which the heart forces blood through the blood vessels.

Increased heart rate
To beat faster and pump more blood, the heart muscle needs an increase in its supply of blood. This blood reaches the heart muscle via the coronary arteries.

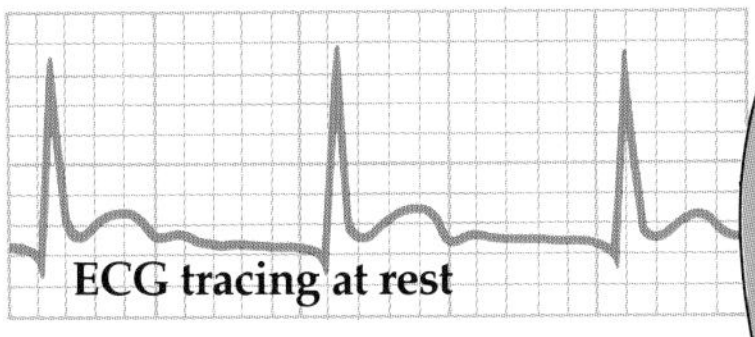

ECG tracing at rest

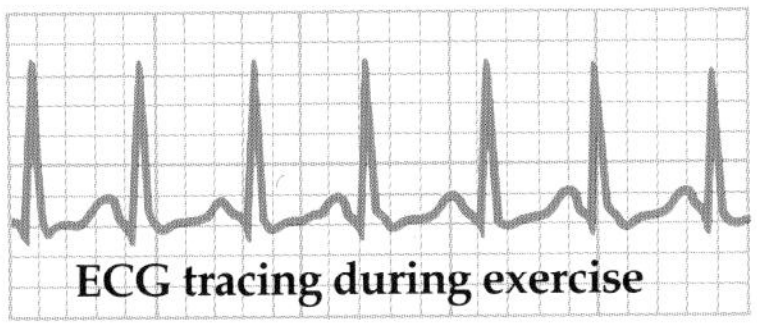

ECG tracing during exercise

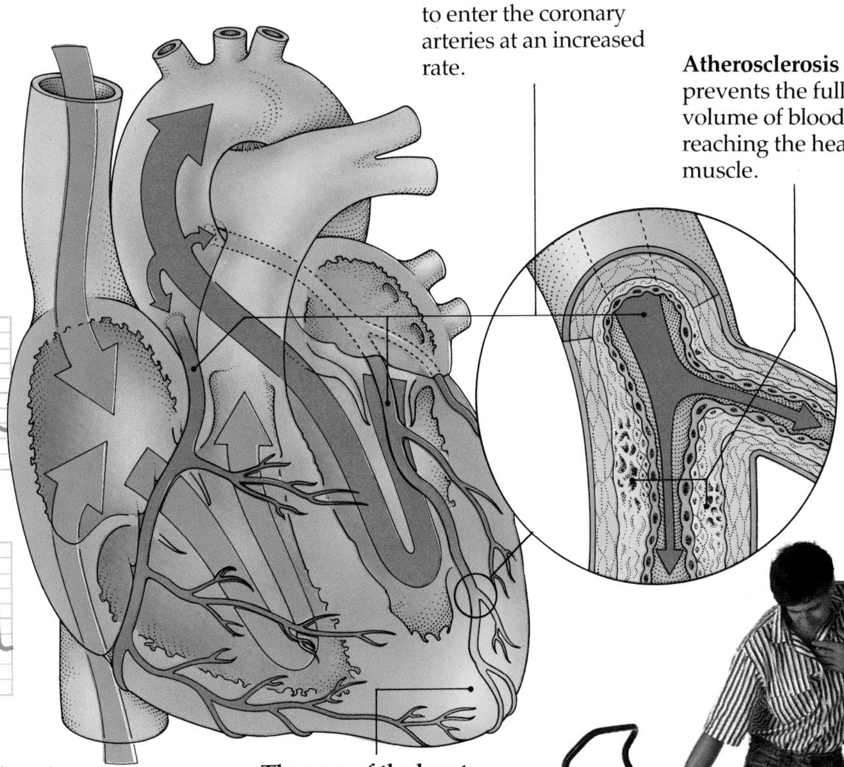

Exercise causes blood to enter the coronary arteries at an increased rate.

Atherosclerosis prevents the full volume of blood from reaching the heart muscle.

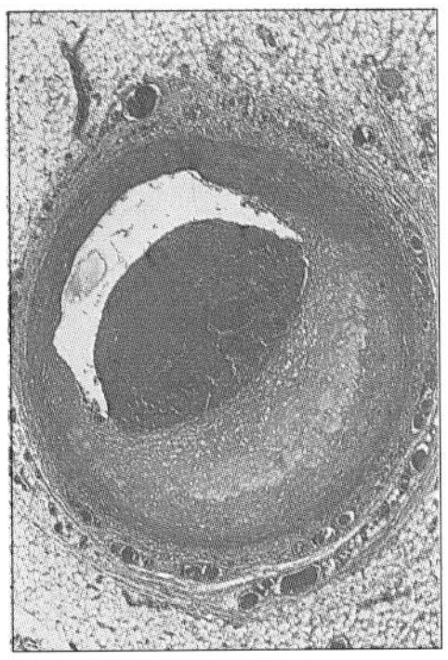

Atherosclerosis
Atherosclerotic narrowing in a coronary artery (left) usually allows enough blood to get to the heart at rest. However, during exercise, the narrowing can prevent an adequate supply of blood from making its way through the coronary circulation.

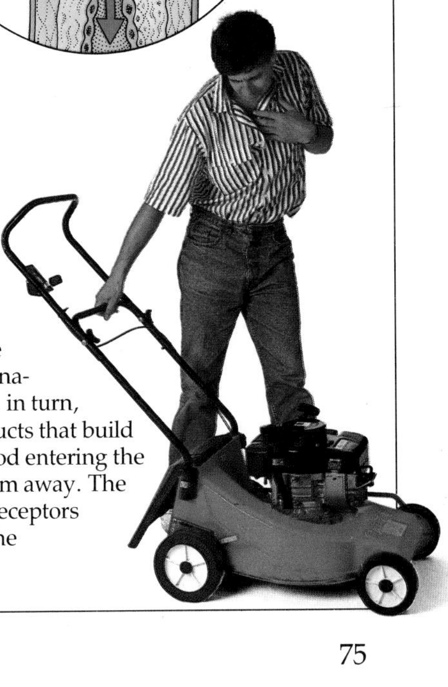

The area of the heart supplied by the narrowed artery suffers from a depleted blood supply. Starved of adequate oxygen and glucose, the heart provides energy by alternative chemical processes. They, in turn, produce chemical waste products that build up because the amount of blood entering the area is insufficient to carry them away. The waste chemicals trigger pain receptors in the heart muscle, causing the severe pain of angina.

ing intensity. There may be a burning sensation, a feeling of choking or as if a great weight were resting on the chest, or a sense of extreme tiredness. The arms may feel very heavy.

When does angina occur?

Angina is almost always brought on by exertion. After the exertion is stopped, it usually lasts for only a few minutes. Less effort may be required to produce angina soon after a meal, if you are anxious or angry, or if you are in a cold wind. Because the pattern of angina is usually constant for an individual, any change for the worse in this pattern is a cause for concern. If the attacks become more frequent, longer in duration, or occur during milder exertion or at rest, angina is described as "unstable." In up to one third of cases, unstable angina leads to a heart attack within 3 months.

How is angina treated?

Angina can be relieved dramatically by treatment with nitrate drugs (see page 130), beta blockers (see page 129), or calcium channel blockers (see page 132). Sometimes surgery is performed to bypass a narrowed coronary artery (see CORONARY ARTERY BYPASS SURGERY on page 78) or to widen an artery (see BALLOON ANGIOPLASTY on page 118).

Narrowed arteries
In this color-enhanced angiogram of the coronary blood supply, the effects of atherosclerosis are clearly visible. In the center of the photograph, healthy sections of the left coronary artery, where the blood supply is not obstructed, appear as wide, pink ribbons. However, at top right, atherosclerosis has reduced the diameter of certain sections, and the blood flow through them is restricted.

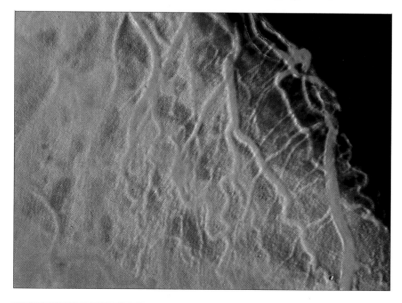

Q Although I stay carefully within the exercise limits recommended by my doctor, my angina attacks still surprise me. Are there other factors I should know about?

A The point at which you feel your angina beginning can be affected by several factors, including the temperature and whether you have been smoking recently or have eaten a heavy meal. Angina is usually worse in cold weather and may be triggered by going from a warm room out into the cold air. Also, walking into a strong wind reduces the distance you can walk before the angina starts.

Q My uncle seldom exerts himself, yet he still suffers from angina attacks. Why is this?

A Attacks of angina can occur at rest in people whose coronary arteries are severely diseased, but may also occur as a result of spasm of the coronary arteries, sometimes produced by stress or for unknown reasons. Angina that is present when you awaken is often preceded by a violent dream that has temporarily raised the heart rate and the blood pressure.

Q I had my first angina attack a few weeks ago. How often should I expect them in the future?

A Angina attacks vary in frequency from several each day to occasional attacks separated by weeks, months, or even years. The severity of the angina may remain constant for years or may increase progressively. Sometimes, if new arterial channels open up in the heart muscle, angina disappears altogether. In other cases, angina disappears when a segment of heart muscle dies after a heart attack.

MONITOR YOUR SYMPTOMS
CHEST PAIN

A sudden pain in the chest can be alarming and often causes people to believe that they are having a heart attack. Although heart attacks are not uncommon – more than 1.5 million Americans have one every year – there are many other, less serious causes of chest pain.

WARNING

The warning signs of a heart attack are:

◆ Crushing central chest pain, unrelieved by rest, that may radiate down the left arm or up the neck and jaw.
◆ Weakness and sweating.
◆ A feeling of impending doom.
◆ Nausea and sometimes vomiting.

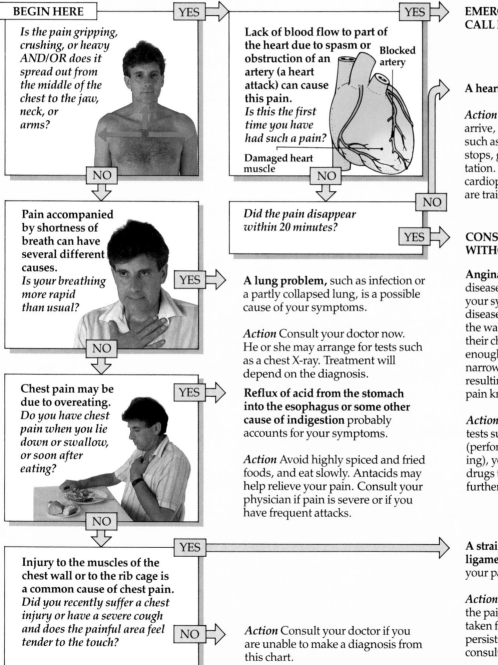

BEGIN HERE

Is the pain gripping, crushing, or heavy AND/OR does it spread out from the middle of the chest to the jaw, neck, or arms?

YES

Lack of blood flow to part of the heart due to spasm or obstruction of an artery (a heart attack) can cause this pain.
Is this the first time you have had such a pain?

Blocked artery

Damaged heart muscle

YES

**EMERGENCY
CALL FOR MEDICAL HELP NOW!**

A heart attack is possible

Action While you wait for help to arrive, loosen any tight clothing, such as collars or belts. If breathing stops, give mouth-to-mouth resuscitation. If there is no pulse, perform cardiopulmonary resuscitation if you are trained to do so.

NO

NO

Did the pain disappear within 20 minutes?

NO

YES

Pain accompanied by shortness of breath can have several different causes.
Is your breathing more rapid than usual?

YES

A lung problem, such as infection or a partly collapsed lung, is a possible cause of your symptoms.

Action Consult your doctor now. He or she may arrange for tests such as a chest X-ray. Treatment will depend on the diagnosis.

**CONSULT YOUR DOCTOR
WITHOUT DELAY!**

Angina due to coronary heart disease is a possible explanation for your symptoms. In coronary heart disease, fatty deposits accumulate in the walls of the arteries, narrowing their channels. During exercise, not enough oxygen can get through the narrowed vessels to the heart muscle, resulting in the characteristic chest pain known as angina.

Action If angina is diagnosed after tests such as electrocardiography (performed while you are exercising), your doctor will prescribe drugs to help prevent and relieve further attacks.

NO

Chest pain may be due to overeating.
Do you have chest pain when you lie down or swallow, or soon after eating?

YES

Reflux of acid from the stomach into the esophagus or some other cause of indigestion probably accounts for your symptoms.

Action Avoid highly spiced and fried foods, and eat slowly. Antacids may help relieve your pain. Consult your physician if pain is severe or if you have frequent attacks.

NO

YES

A strained or bruised muscle or ligament is the most likely cause of your pain.

Action Avoid strenuous activity until the pain subsides. Painkillers may be taken for relief. However, if pain persists for more than a few days, consult your doctor.

Injury to the muscles of the chest wall or to the rib cage is a common cause of chest pain.
Did you recently suffer a chest injury or have a severe cough and does the painful area feel tender to the touch?

NO

Action Consult your doctor if you are unable to make a diagnosis from this chart.

SURGICAL PROCEDURES
CORONARY ARTERY BYPASS SURGERY

URGERY MAY BE RECOMMENDED when a person continues to have angina at rest despite maximum drug treatment. Coronary artery bypass employing a portion of the saphenous vein (below) or the internal mammary artery (far right) is a well-established procedure that can be performed to restore a healthy blood supply to the heart muscle. The object of both procedures is to relieve angina and reduce the chances of a heart attack. Both operations require the use of a heart-lung machine (right). Balloon angioplasty (see page 118) is a newer, alternative technique that is used to stretch open a narrowed coronary artery or other narrowed artery in the body.

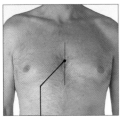

Incision

1 After administration of a general anesthetic, an incision is made down the center of the breastbone, the chest is opened, and the heart is exposed by opening the pericardium.

2 Incisions are made in the leg, and a length of saphenous vein for use in the bypass is removed.

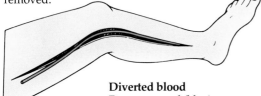

Diverted blood
Deoxygenated (blue) blood is diverted to the machine by means of tubes inserted via cannulas into the patient's venae cavae.

THE HEART-LUNG MACHINE

Any time surgery is performed on the interior or exterior of the heart, requiring the heart to be stopped, a cardiopulmonary bypass machine (heart-lung machine) must be connected to the patient to take over the function of the heart and lungs. Deoxygenated (blue) blood returning to the right side of the patient's heart is diverted to the machine.

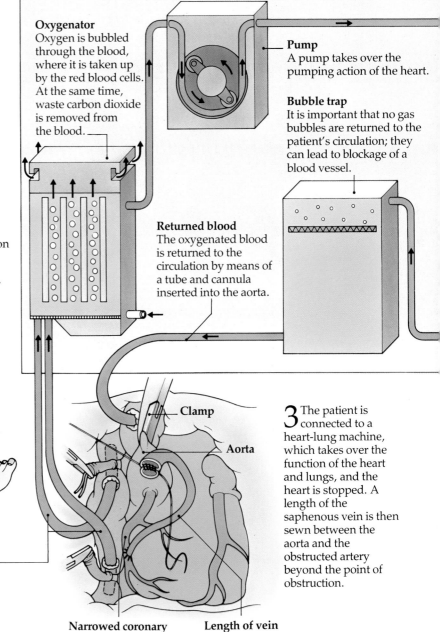

Oxygenator
Oxygen is bubbled through the blood, where it is taken up by the red blood cells. At the same time, waste carbon dioxide is removed from the blood.

Pump
A pump takes over the pumping action of the heart.

Bubble trap
It is important that no gas bubbles are returned to the patient's circulation; they can lead to blockage of a blood vessel.

Returned blood
The oxygenated blood is returned to the circulation by means of a tube and cannula inserted into the aorta.

Clamp

Aorta

Narrowed coronary artery

Length of vein

3 The patient is connected to a heart-lung machine, which takes over the function of the heart and lungs, and the heart is stopped. A length of the saphenous vein is then sewn between the aorta and the obstructed artery beyond the point of obstruction.

Bypassing the heart
The heart-lung machine (right and below) oxygenates, filters, and cools or warms the blood, removes any bubbles from it, and pumps the blood back into the person's aorta for distribution to the body.

INTERNAL MAMMARY ARTERY BYPASS

An alternative to vein bypass is to use one or both of a pair of arteries that run down the inside of the chest wall – the internal mammary arteries – as a bypass.

1 The lower end of an internal mammary artery can be freed from smaller arteries that branch from it to supply the chest wall.

Obstructed coronary artery

Internal mammary artery

Filter
The filter removes any tiny particles that may have been introduced into the blood from the machine.

2 The internal mammary artery is then moved backward and connected to one of the coronary arteries beyond the narrowed area. Alternatively, doctors may take sections of arteries from the upper abdomen for use in bypass surgery.

Internal mammery artery used as bypass

Heat exchanger
This cools the blood before it is returned to the patient, lowering the body temperature and allowing more time to perform the operation. Afterward, the heat exchanger warms the blood, and thus the patient.

Aorta

4 A triple bypass is shown at left and in the photograph at right. After the bypass, blood can flow from the aorta around the obstructions in the affected arteries and on to the heart muscle.

ight oronary rtery

Circumflex branch of left coronary artery

Left anterior descending artery

5 The heart is then restarted, the heart-lung machine is disconnected, and the patient's chest is closed.

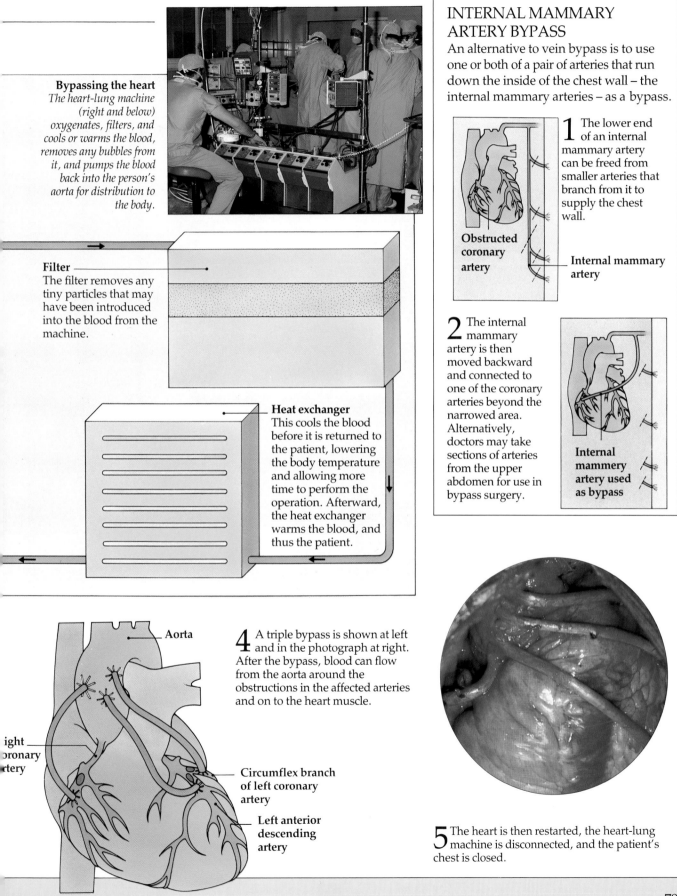

LIVING WITH ANGINA

If you suffer from angina, it is important that you understand this symptom and the factors that bring on an attack in your case. There are also steps you can take to keep the influence of angina on your life to a minimum.

 Smoking. Of all the preventive measures you can take, none is more important than quitting smoking completely and permanently. To put it bluntly, if you continue to smoke cigarettes when you have angina, your behavior borders on being suicidal.

 Obesity. Losing weight if you are overweight will help improve your condition. In some overweight people, losing weight is all that is necessary to eliminate the angina altogether. Staying trim also reduces the work your heart must perform.

 Coffee. Cut your caffeine intake to no more than two cups of coffee or other caffeine-containing drinks every day. You might also consider switching to a decaffeinated substitute.

 Diet. Change your diet to one containing plenty of fiber – whole-grain cereals, fruit, peas, beans, lentils, and fresh vegetables. Eat much less fatty meat and fewer high-fat dairy products, which contain cholesterol and saturated fats.

 Blood pressure. You must have your blood pressure checked every time you visit your doctor. If your blood pressure is high, it is vital that it be treated. Even a small rise above the normal level in the diastolic pressure places additional strain on your heart, which may lead to a heart attack.

 Exercise. You can, through the use of exercise that does not provoke angina, improve the efficiency of your heart and muscles so that your capacity for exercise increases. Some doctors believe that you can exercise beyond the point of onset of pain ("walking through angina") but this is controversial. Other doctors believe that there is no reason to challenge yourself in this way and risk having a heart attack in the process. There is no doubt, however, that regular, sustained exercise, such as walking or swimming, can increase your exercise tolerance and improve your quality of life.

 Know your limits. Be aware of the amount of activity you can perform before you experience angina. This is important so that you can recognize any suggestion that your condition is worsening. If anything odd or unusually severe regarding the distribution, severity, or duration of the pain occurs during your routine exercise program, alert your doctor and ask someone to drive you to your doctor's office or to a hospital immediately.

 Medication. Never try to do without your nitroglycerin in the mistaken belief that regular use of this drug will cause it to lose its effect. Anything that eliminates your angina is good for you. Don't be frightened to use nitroglycerin many times a day, if necessary. The worst consequence of doing so may be the development of a headache. Also, do not abruptly stop taking beta blockers or other antianginal medicines.

Storage. Remember that excessive exposure to air, heat, or moisture can cause nitroglycerin to lose its potency. At home, keep your tablets in a tightly sealed container and don't purchase too many at one time. Replace your "carry-around" supply every 6 weeks.

HOW DANGEROUS IS ANGINA?

If you have angina, the outlook depends on a variety of factors, such as gender, age, and whether or not you once smoked or still do. However, the outlook depends primarily on how seriously your coronary arteries are affected. In the chart (right), the outlook for several types of male angina sufferers is compared in terms of relative life expectancy.

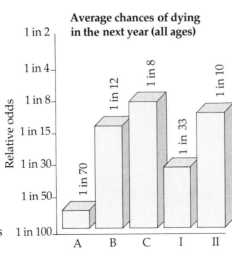

Average chances of dying in the next year (all ages)

Relative odds

1 in 2
1 in 4
1 in 8
1 in 15
1 in 30
1 in 50
1 in 100

A — 1 in 70
B — 1 in 12
C — 1 in 8
I — 1 in 33
II — 1 in 10

Type of angina sufferer

A No history of heart attacks, a normal ECG at rest, and normal blood pressure

B No history of heart attacks and either an abnormal ECG or high blood pressure

C No history of heart attacks, but both an abnormal ECG and high blood pressure

I One coronary artery affected by atherosclerosis

II Three coronary arteries affected by atherosclerosis

CASE HISTORY
SUDDEN CHEST PAIN

AFTER DONALD ATTENDED a board meeting, the elevator was delayed. Unwilling to wait, he sprinted upstairs. Just as Donald entered his office, he felt a burning pain in his chest, which spread up to his neck and down his left arm. Although the pain soon disappeared, Donald was alarmed and he resolved to see his doctor that same day.

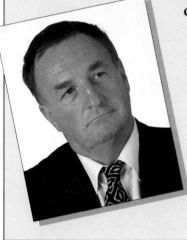

PERSONAL DETAILS
Name Donald Cameron
Age 57
Occupation Investment banker
Family Donald's mother is well at 81, but his father died at 60 of heart disease.

MEDICAL BACKGROUND
Donald is quiet and seemingly relaxed, but he is, in fact, extremely ambitious. He is suspicious of his colleagues and represses his hostility toward them. His doctor has expressed concern about his blood pressure on several occasions. Donald's attempts to quit smoking have been unsuccessful, and he tends to be a little overweight.

THE CONSULTATION
Donald tells his doctor that he was convinced that he was dying of a heart attack, but the pain had disappeared within a few minutes and he had felt much better. The doctor listens to Donald's heart, takes an electrocardiogram (ECG), which is normal, and arranges for him to have an exercise ECG and a blood test to check his cholesterol level.

FURTHER INVESTIGATION
The results of several tests on Donald's cholesterol level are normal. However, analysis of his exercise ECG reveals an abnormality characteristic of coronary artery insufficiency (inadequate blood flow to the heart to meet increased demand).

Learning to relax
After undergoing the balloon angioplasty operation to widen his obstructed coronary artery, Donald took up yoga to help relax, quit smoking completely, and is learning more effective ways of coping with his emotions.

THE DOCTOR'S IMPRESSION
Donald's doctor believes that Donald has had an attack of angina. The circumstances under which he experienced the angina may have been exceptional and there is a chance that it may not recur.

The doctor does not prescribe any treatment, but Donald is given some nitroglycerin tablets to use if the angina should recur. He is urged to quit smoking and to lose some weight and is advised to return weekly for blood pressure checks.

THE FOLLOW-UP
Three weeks after his first attack, Donald tries some brisk walking. After walking about 200 yards he has another angina attack, this one less severe, that disappears within 2 or 3 minutes. Donald decides to give up his brisk walking but is shocked, 2 days later, when he feels the angina again while walking uphill at a relaxed pace.

THE DIAGNOSIS
Donald's doctor is concerned and suspects that he may have UNSTABLE ANGINA. He discusses his suspicions with Donald and recommends that he have a coronary angiogram. The angiogram shows a severe narrowing high on the front branch of Donald's left coronary artery, although the artery below the obstruction appears to be healthy.

THE TREATMENT
Balloon angioplasty is performed, and Donald's symptoms do not return. His doctor explains to him that smoking, stress, and bottled-up hostility contributed to the development of the atherosclerosis that narrowed his coronary artery and caused the angina. The doctor recommends some methods of preventing a recurrence.

HEART ATTACK

Potentially more serious than the narrowing of a coronary artery by atherosclerosis is the tendency of atheromatous plaques to rupture and promote the formation of blood clots. Any blood clot that forms on top of a plaque can block the artery altogether, cutting off the blood supply to a part of the heart.

A heart attack occurs when an area of the heart muscle is so severely deprived of blood that it can no longer survive. This is a myocardial infarction ("myo" means muscle, "cardio" means relating to the heart, and "infarct" is a wedge-shaped area of dead tissue caused by obstruction of the artery supplying it).

When do heart attacks occur?

Heart attacks tend to occur with little or no warning other than, in some cases, a feeling of fatigue. Unlike angina, a heart attack usually does not take place during times of exertion, although it is not uncommon for a heart attack to occur just afterward. This may be because the blood clots that cause myocardial infarctions tend to form when the flow through the artery is sluggish.

What are the chances of survival?

In 1989, 8 to 15 percent of heart attack victims who reached the hospital died within 3 weeks. When thrombolytic (clot-dissolving) drugs (see page 137) were given within 3 to 4 hours after the heart attack, the mortality dropped substantially. Elderly people do less well than the young and the middle aged. Those who die within several days after the heart attack almost always have a blockage high in a coronary artery or inside a large branch of the artery.

EMERGENCY ACTION

If you think you are having a heart attack, or if you see someone collapse and suspect a heart problem, have someone call an ambulance immediately. Time is vital; most deaths from cardiac arrest after a heart attack occur very soon after the attack. Most can be prevented through speedy medical intervention to restore the heartbeat and rhythm. While waiting for help to arrive, loosen any tight clothing around the chest and neck and keep the victim as calm as possible. If the victim becomes unconscious, check for signs of breathing and a pulse. If there are no signs of breathing or a pulse, and you are trained in cardio-pulmonary resuscitation (CPR), begin CPR immediately. Otherwise, call for help.

WHAT ARE THE SYMPTOMS AND SIGNS OF A HEART ATTACK?

Fever
Within 12 hours of a heart attack there is almost always a fever. The fever usually subsides within 4 or 5 days but occasionally lasts for a week.

Radiating pain
In almost 70 percent of cases, the pain radiates to the neck and jaw, and usually down the left arm. There may be heaviness or tingling in one or both arms.

Chest pain
More than 80 percent of heart attack victims suffer pain in the chest. The pain tends to be described as crushing or choking in nature, similar to that of angina but usually more severe. It usually lasts for at least 20 minutes and does not cease during rest.

Breathlessness
There may be breathlessness when lying down that is relieved only by standing or sitting upright. In addition, breathing may be difficult or labored.

Other symptoms
Sweating and belching up air are common. There may be nausea, dizziness, or faintness.

HOW DOES A BLOCKED BLOOD SUPPLY AFFECT THE HEART?

Death of a segment of heart muscle does not necessarily mean death for its owner. The outcome depends on the amount of muscle affected and the state of the arteries supplying the surrounding heart muscle.

Often, the surrounding, partially damaged heart muscle continues to work, sometimes at a lower level of efficiency. This gives time for a healing scar to form and for the heart to recover most of its structural strength.

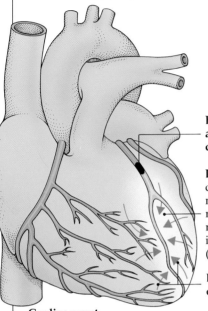

Blockage in left anterior descending coronary artery

Left ventricle is deprived of blood. The muscle fibers undergo random excitation, resulting in rapid and irregular contractions (fibrillation)

Direction of contractions

Cardiac arrest
In rare cases, a blockage stops the heart muscle's action altogether (asystole) or replaces it with a useless, fluttering contraction of the large lower chambers (ventricular fibrillation). Both of these conditions are called cardiac arrest. Ventricular fibrillation may also occur in the absence of a recent heart attack.

Right coronary artery

Arterial branches

Blockages at arterial ends

Fibrosis caused by nutrient depletion

"Small" heart attack
If a tiny end branch of an artery is blocked, a small segment of heart muscle – much less than its full thickness – may die. With atherosclerosis of the smaller vessels, patchy scarring can occur, sometimes without symptoms of a heart attack. Ultimately, this results in deterioration in the functional efficiency of the heart.

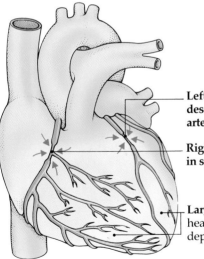

Left anterior descending coronary artery in spasm

Right coronary artery in spasm

Large areas of the heart muscle are deprived of blood

Coronary spasm
In addition to blockage of the coronary arteries by a blood clot, cardiac arrest can also be caused by coronary spasm. For reasons not fully understood, the coronary arteries can go into spasm, closing off the blood supply long enough to stop the heart.

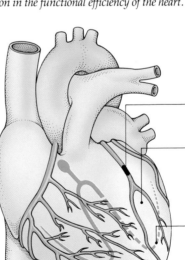

Blockage in left anterior descending coronary artery

Left ventricle is deprived of blood

Electrical impulses cannot pass through the damaged tissue, so the contractions of the left ventricle cease to be coordinated with those of the other chambers of the heart

Heart block
If part of the heart's electrical conducting system is damaged, the condition known as heart block may result. In this disorder, the passage of the electrical impulse from the upper part of the heart is not conveyed, as usual, to the ventricles.

More than half of those who die of a heart attack do so within 1 or 2 hours after the onset of symptoms. Ironically, many people who die suddenly in this way, although invariably showing extensive atherosclerosis, often show no sign of any recent blockage of an artery or death of muscle tissue. The cause of death may be an acute spasm of the coronary arteries or an irregular heart rhythm that is related to some previous damage to the heart. Many of these people could be saved if given prompt cardiopulmonary resuscitation.

What is the outlook for survivors?

The outlook during the first few hours after a heart attack depends on the degree to which the performance of the heart has been reduced and on whether any severe rhythm disturbances develop. If the damaged area is large, there is a risk that the main pumping chambers of the heart, especially on the left side, will be unable to pump strongly enough to maintain the circulation. This is called heart failure. A rapid, weak heart action, low blood pressure, and reduced formation of urine are other warning signs of heart failure.

Victims of heart attack who show no evidence of heart failure 48 hours afterward, who do not have a rapid or irregular pulse, and whose conduction pathways of the heart seem unaffected, are likely to recover and often are discharged from the hospital within a week.

Is there any treatment?

A major recent advance in treatment was the discovery that, if the enzyme streptokinase is introduced into the coronary arteries through a catheter, arteries blocked by clotting can be reopened in up to 80 percent of cases. The artery must

HOW MANY PEOPLE SURVIVE A HEART ATTACK?

If the total number of people suffering a heart attack at 1 AM on January 1, 1990 were taken as a representative sample, a statistical analysis would indicate that the fate of those people would be as shown in the chart below. However, the chances of survival vary considerably from person to person according to factors such as age, gender, and whether or not the person has diabetes.

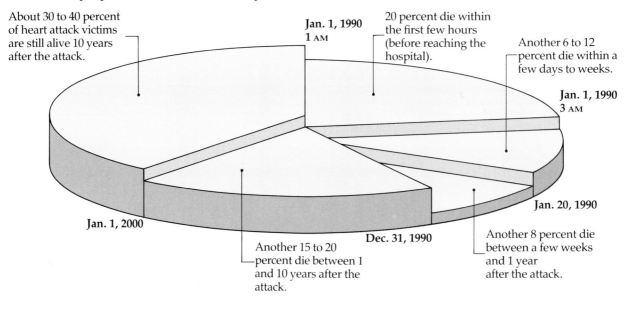

About 30 to 40 percent of heart attack victims are still alive 10 years after the attack.

Jan. 1, 1990
1 AM

20 percent die within the first few hours (before reaching the hospital).

Another 6 to 12 percent die within a few days to weeks.

Jan. 1, 1990
3 AM

Jan. 1, 2000

Jan. 20, 1990

Dec. 31, 1990

Another 15 to 20 percent die between 1 and 10 years after the attack.

Another 8 percent die between a few weeks and 1 year after the attack.

LIFE AFTER A HEART ATTACK

In the past, if you had a heart attack, doctors advised you to rest in bed for 6 weeks and restrict your physical activities for at least another 6 weeks. Today, doctors believe that this approach is ultimately harmful, and that a gradual, but determined, attempt to regain your physical capacity is the best medicine. Patients are encouraged to get out of bed within a few days. Eliminating factors in your life-style that may have contributed to the heart attack is another important way to minimize the risk of having another one.

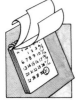 **Work.** Depending upon your occupation, after a minor heart attack you might expect to be back at work within a month. After a more serious heart attack, it may take about 3 months. A period of part-time work before resuming full activity is sometimes recommended.

 Stress. Keep your work schedule within reasonable limits and avoid those situations that you know are stressful. Learn to delegate more of your work. Do not take on more than you can handle. Find a relaxing hobby and make time for other leisurely activities.

 Alcohol. There is good evidence that a moderate alcohol intake – two daily drinks of whisky (1 ounce each), wine (4 ounces each), or beer (12 ounces each) – is not harmful to your heart. Avoid heavy drinking because of its effect on your liver, heart, and weight.

 Insurance. Inform your insurance company of your heart attack if you are applying for a new policy. Coverage may extend to include cardiac rehabilitation programs, which have not been proven to enhance survival, but probably add to the quality of life.

 Sex. There is no reason why your normal pattern of sexual relations should not be resumed about 3 to 4 weeks after a heart attack, unless your doctor advises against it. Although sexual intercourse raises your blood pressure and pulse rate, most hearts can tolerate the stress.

 Medication. There is evidence that taking aspirin regularly is a valuable measure in preventing recurrence of a heart attack and an initial heart attack in men over 50. The amount and frequency is controversial but most experts would agree with one 325 mg tablet every other day.

 Retirement. The evidence suggests that, if you are able to work, retiring simply because you have had a heart attack is medically and psychologically a bad choice. The work environment may also help you overcome any depression more quickly.

 Exercise. Swim regularly. Swimming three times a week, working to increase the distance each time, is ideal. A brisk walking program for 20 or 30 minutes three times a week provides similar benefits. Make sure that you stay within reasonable limits of breathlessness.

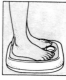 **Obesity.** Ask your doctor to recommend a 1,500-calorie diet if you are a man or 1,200-calorie diet if you are a woman. When you reach your desired weight, it should be possible to increase your diet to about 2,200 calories (for men) or 1,800 to 2,000 (for women).

 Cigarettes. Quit smoking. This is probably the single most important factor in decreasing your risk of having another heart attack. Nicotine chewing gum and behavior modification programs are useful adjuncts to the most important factor – your desire to quit.

be unblocked within 4 hours of closure; otherwise, the heart muscle it serves will die. Arterial catheterization, which allows the doctor to instill the enzyme directly, is a specialized technique available only in some hospitals.

Streptokinase, and other thrombolytic drugs such as tissue plasminogen activator, may also be infused into a vein. This technique is available in most hospitals and even outside the hospital. When administered into a vein instead of directly into the obstructed coronary artery, the drugs are diluted and their effects may be reduced. About 60 percent of blocked arteries can be opened by giving the drugs continuously for periods of 30 to 60 minutes within 3 to 4 hours after the blockage has occurred. However, there is a risk of internal bleeding and stroke, particularly in the elderly and in people who have hypertension.

Research is underway to determine the optimum choice, dosage, and method of administering these life-saving drugs.

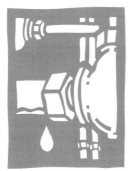

HEART VALVE DISORDERS

THE EFFICIENCY OF THE HEART as a pump depends not only on the force of its contractions but also on the correct functioning of its four valves. The valves are subject to a variety of disorders – most commonly the failure to open or close properly. A serious valve disorder can have a progressively debilitating effect that can ultimately be fatal unless surgery is performed to correct the problem.

The heart has four valves. Two of them are situated between the upper and lower chambers (atrium and ventricle) on each side of the heart – the tricuspid valve on the right and the mitral valve on the left. The other two lie at the exit of each ventricle into the two large arteries carrying blood from the heart – the pulmonary valve at the exit from the right ventricle into the pulmonary artery, and the aortic valve at the exit from the left ventricle into the aorta.

HOW THE VALVES WORK

The valves allow blood to pass into and out of the heart chambers in one direction only, with no backflow of blood. They consist of cupped, or bowl-shaped, segments called cusps. When blood is moving in the right direction, the cusps separate widely; when blood tries to move in the opposite direction, the cusps close tightly and form a watertight seal.

THE MOVEMENT OF BLOOD

When the ventricles contract, the pulmonary and aortic valves open to let blood out of the heart. Between heartbeats, the ventricles relax and the aortic and pulmonary valves close. The tricuspid and mitral valves then open to allow blood to pass into the heart from the body tissues and lungs.

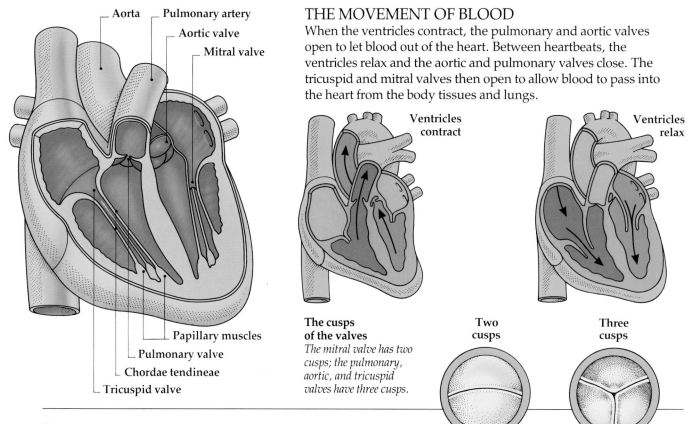

Aorta — Pulmonary artery

Aortic valve

Mitral valve

Ventricles contract

Ventricles relax

Papillary muscles

Pulmonary valve

Chordae tendineae

Tricuspid valve

The cusps of the valves
The mitral valve has two cusps; the pulmonary, aortic, and tricuspid valves have three cusps.

Two cusps

Three cusps

Opening and closing

The opening and closing of the valves is brought about by movement of blood and by constantly changing differences in pressure on either side of the valves.

The mitral and tricuspid valves are subject to considerable pressure when the powerful lower chambers (ventricles) contract. To prevent the cusps of the valves from ballooning upward into the atria under this pressure, they are connected by strong fibrous cords (called chordae tendineae) to short, fingerlike muscles (called papillary muscles) rising from the floors of the ventricles. The papillary muscles contract and tense the cords when the valves close.

The aortic and pulmonary valves, which are smaller and have more rigid cusps than the other two valves, are less liable to be pushed backward out of position under pressure, so they do not require the same fastening mechanism.

TYPES OF DISORDERS

Valve disorders fall into two principal groups. The first includes disorders in which a valve is narrowed or fails to open properly, obstructing the forward flow of blood. This is called stenosis, and usually occurs when the affected valves have become inflamed or calcified. It may also occur as a congenital defect (see CONGENITAL HEART DISEASE on page 68).

The second group of valve disorders includes those in which the valves fail to close properly, causing a backward leakage, or regurgitation, of blood. These valves are called incompetent or insufficient. Backward leakage of blood may result from coronary heart disease, from rheumatic heart disease, or from bacterial endocarditis.

Of the four valves, those on the left side of the heart – the aortic and mitral valves – are more commonly affected by disorders because the more powerful contractions of the left ventricle place a greater strain on these two valves.

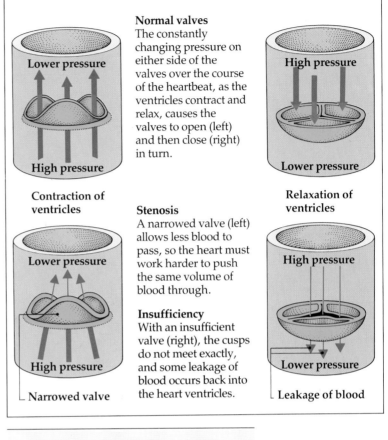

THE AORTIC AND PULMONARY VALVES

Normal valves
The constantly changing pressure on either side of the valves over the course of the heartbeat, as the ventricles contract and relax, causes the valves to open (left) and then close (right) in turn.

Lower pressure

High pressure

High pressure

Lower pressure

Contraction of ventricles

Relaxation of ventricles

Stenosis
A narrowed valve (left) allows less blood to pass, so the heart must work harder to push the same volume of blood through.

Insufficiency
With an insufficient valve (right), the cusps do not meet exactly, and some leakage of blood occurs back into the heart ventricles.

Lower pressure

High pressure

High pressure

Lower pressure

Narrowed valve

Leakage of blood

THE AORTIC VALVE

The aortic valve may fail to open properly (stenosis) or may fail to close properly (insufficiency or regurgitation).

Aortic stenosis

This is the most common heart valve disorder in the US. It affects men more often than women. Aortic stenosis may be present from birth, may be secondary to degeneration of the cusps of the valve from unknown causes, or may result from rheumatic heart disease.

Narrowing of the valve channel limits the heart's output. The extra work required to pump blood through a narrowed outlet leads to enlargement of the left ventricle. There are few, if any, symptoms resulting from aortic stenosis until age 50. When symptoms occur, they usually include breathlessness during exertion, faintness, and angina.

Heart failure is treated with drugs such as digitalis. Restriction of salt and the use of diuretics (drugs that encourage the loss of fluid from the body) reduce excessive amounts of retained body fluids.

A major decision is whether or not surgery is needed and, if so, when. Heart valve replacement (see page 89) always carries some risk, but it can produce a remarkable improvement. Balloon valvuloplasty (widening a narrowed valve by means of a balloon catheter introduced into the heart) has been successfully used on an investigational basis, but the length of time the stenosis is relieved by this procedure remains to be determined.

Aortic insufficiency

Aortic insufficiency is a less common heart valve disorder that places considerable strain on the left ventricle, causing it to thicken and enlarge. To eject the volume of blood required by the body, the rise in blood pressure with each heart contraction is much higher than normal. But, because blood can flow back into the heart, the pressure then collapses to an unusually low level. This "collapsing pulse" is a feature of aortic insufficiency.

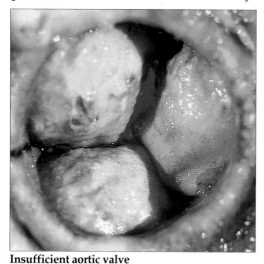

Insufficient aortic valve
The aortic valve opens to let blood out of the heart into the lungs and body tissues. An insufficient valve, such as the surgically removed valve shown above, does not close properly. It places strain on the heart by permitting blood to re-enter the heart (instead of moving into the circulation) after it has been ejected.

TYPES OF REPLACEMENT VALVES

Mechanical (metal and plastic) valves include the Starr-Edwards caged-ball valve and the Bjork-Shiley tilting disc valve. They are durable, but tend to encourage the formation of blood clots, so the patient must undergo long-term therapy with anticoagulant drugs. Biological valves include the Carpentier-Edwards valve, which is a modified pig valve (pigs have the same size hearts as humans). Biological valves are less durable, but don't require the use of anticoagulants.

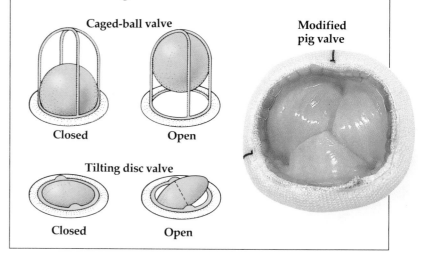

Caged-ball valve

Modified pig valve

Closed   Open

Tilting disc valve

Closed   Open

THE MITRAL VALVE

The mitral valve can be affected by both stenosis and insufficiency.

Mitral stenosis

In established mitral stenosis, the cusps of the valves become thickened and often have deposits of clotted blood (thrombus) on their upper surfaces. The chordae tendineae also may be shortened and stuck together.

Narrowing of the valve diminishes tolerance to exercise and causes breathlessness, fatigue, and heaviness of the limbs. A characteristic sign seen in people with mitral stenosis with rheumatic heart disease is malar flush – a purple-pink tinge to the cheekbones and lips. An associated problem is congestion of blood in the lungs, which encourages both chest infections and the accumulation of fluid in the lungs. This accumulation is known as pulmonary edema. Eventually, heart failure may develop.

DENTAL TREATMENT

Dental work and some invasive diagnostic procedures can be dangerous to people with heart valve disease. Using medical instruments on the teeth or mucous membranes is often followed by a brief period in which bacteria, normally present in these areas, appear in the bloodstream. While this is harmless in healthy people, those with heart valve disease are at risk of a serious condition called endocarditis (see page 63). Antibiotics are given to decrease the risk.

SURGICAL PROCEDURES
HEART VALVE REPLACEMENT

VALVE REPLACEMENT **is the most radical form of treatment for heart valve disease. Though it carries some risks, it can often bring a remarkable improvement in the patient's condition. Replacing a valve requires the use of a heart-lung machine and may take several hours to perform. The steps in surgically replacing a diseased aortic valve with an artificial caged-ball valve are shown below.**

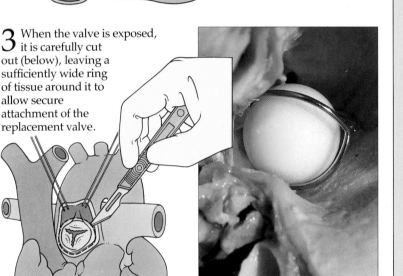

Aorta

Aortic valve

Left ventricle

Repair or replace?
The aortic valve, lying at the exit from the left ventricle of the heart into the aorta, is the heart valve that most commonly requires surgical correction. A narrowed valve can often be widened by means of a balloon catheter, or even a finger, introduced into the left ventricle of the heart while it is still beating. To replace the valve, the heart must be stopped and the aorta itself opened up.

REPLACING AN AORTIC VALVE

1 An incision is made in the breastbone, which is split apart, and the pericardium is cut to gain access to the heart.

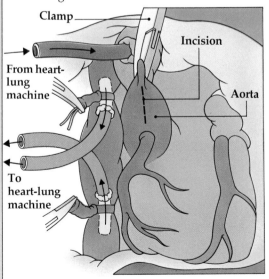

Site of incision

2 The patient is connected to a heart-lung machine, which takes over the function of the heart and lungs. The aorta is clamped and the heart is stopped. An incision is then made in the aorta to gain access to the diseased aortic valve.

Clamp

From heart-lung machine

Incision

Aorta

To heart-lung machine

3 When the valve is exposed, it is carefully cut out (below), leaving a sufficiently wide ring of tissue around it to allow secure attachment of the replacement valve.

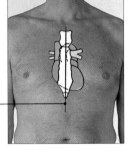

4 The ring of tissue and the sewing ring of the replacement valve are positioned and then stitched securely together (below).

Sutures   New valve

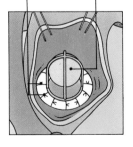

5 Once the new valve is in place (above), the incision in the aorta is sewn closed, the clamp removed, the heart restarted, the heart-lung machine disconnected, and the chest closed. The X-ray below shows a replacement valve in the heart.

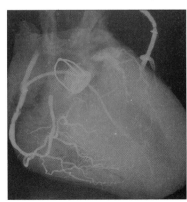

The treatment of mitral stenosis is based on the management of symptoms. Thus, pulmonary edema is treated with diuretics, and chest infections are treated with antibiotics. These drugs do not, however, tackle the basic problem of a narrowed mitral valve channel, which can only be corrected by surgery.

Mitral insufficiency

An insufficient mitral valve can have many causes, the most common one being a condition known as "floppy valve," in which one or both cusps of the valve balloon upward into the atrium. This defect may result from certain rare diseases that affect the body's elastic connective tissues. Some people have a condition known as mitral valve prolapse that is associated with floppy valves, in which case the floppiness appears to increase with age. Other causes of mitral insufficiency include congenital defects in the cusps of the valve, perforation of the valve caused by infection, and shortening of the chordae tendineae by rheumatic heart disease.

Treatment depends on the severity of the disorder. In mild cases, drugs such as diuretics may be used to deal with the effects of moderate heart failure. In severe cases, heart valve replacement is usually necessary.

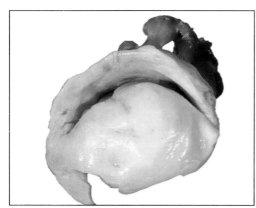

Mitral valve affected by stenosis
Mitral stenosis is almost always associated with the inflammation of the heart that accompanies rheumatic heart disease. The disease is now rare in western countries, although a resurgence in acute rheumatic fever has been reported in some parts of the US.

THE MITRAL VALVE

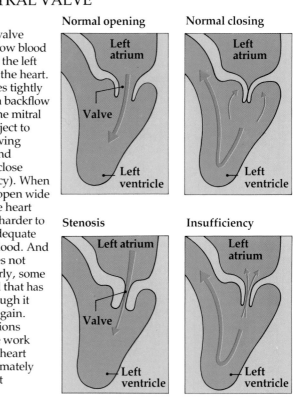

The mitral valve opens to allow blood to pass into the left ventricle of the heart. It then closes tightly to prevent a backflow of blood. The mitral valve is subject to both narrowing (stenosis) and inability to close (insufficiency). When it does not open wide enough, the heart must work harder to pump an adequate supply of blood. And when it does not close properly, some of the blood that has passed through it leaks back again. Both conditions increase the work load on the heart and can ultimately lead to heart failure.

OTHER VALVE DISORDERS

The tricuspid and pulmonary valves on the right side of the heart are less commonly affected by stenosis and insufficiency than those on the left.

The tricuspid valve

Tricuspid insufficiency causes a rise in pressure in the right atrium and in the veins that supply blood to the right atrium. The effect is often mild. In severe cases, congestion can be seen in the neck veins, the liver enlarges, and there is fluid retention throughout the body. The effects of tricuspid stenosis are similar.

The pulmonary valve

A primary disorder of the pulmonary valve is rare, but it may occur as a congenital stenosis or the secondary effect of other heart diseases. Pulmonary insufficiency is a common result of a rise in the blood pressure in the lungs.

RHEUMATIC FEVER

Heart valve disease affects 50 percent of people who have had acute rheumatic fever, a complication of an infection (almost always in the throat) with streptococcal organisms. The causative streptococci carry an antigen (a protein marker on their surfaces) that is identical to a protein found in the heart. Antibodies produced by the body in response to the streptococci proceed to attack parts of the heart, which they misidentify as streptococci.

CASE HISTORY
A STRANGE SENSATION IN THE CHEST

JACK HAS BEEN AWARE for some time that his general energy level has been declining. His legs have felt heavy and his tennis game has been suffering. Jack became mildly concerned a short time ago when he fainted during a tennis game. At the time, he did not think it was important enough to take the time to phone his doctor about it. Then, one afternoon, Jack had a strange sensation in his chest while he was out taking a brisk walk. This prompted him to call his doctor for an appointment.

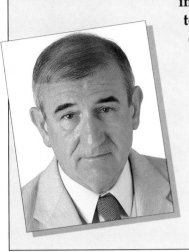

PERSONAL DETAILS
Name Jack Dziedzic
Age 60
Occupation Salesman
Family Jack's parents both died when they were in their 80s.

THE CONSULTATION

The doctor notes, merely by feeling Jack's chest for the heartbeat, that his heart is markedly enlarged. He can feel a vibration through his chest wall during one part of the heart's contraction. The doctor listens with a stethoscope and hears a rough, low-pitched, rasping murmur high up on Jack's chest, just to the right of the middle of his chest. The doctor suspects an aortic valve problem. He orders tests, including an electrocardiogram and an echocardiogram.

The operation
Once Jack's heart valve disorder had been diagnosed, it was quickly decided that a valve replacement operation was the best solution. During the course of the operation, Jack's body was cooled to a temperature of around 68°F (20°C). This permitted surgery with less strain on the brain, liver, and kidneys caused by the interruption to the circulation while Jack was on the heart-lung machine.

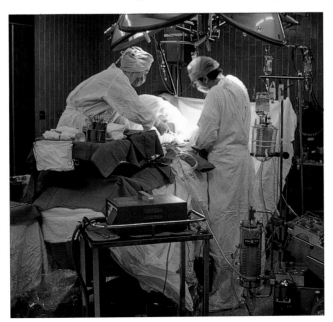

FURTHER INVESTIGATION

The electrocardiogram confirms an enlargement of the left ventricle (pumping chamber) of Jack's heart. The echocardiogram shows obvious signs of deposition of calcium in the aortic valve.

The doctor tells Jack that he considers cardiac catheterization and coronary angiography – an X-ray examination of Jack's coronary arteries using a dye opaque to X-rays – necessary to rule out coronary heart disease as a possible cause of Jack's symptoms. The angiogram images show that Jack's coronary arteries are in excellent condition, but they also reveal a narrow stream of radiopaque dye passing through Jack's aortic valve.

THE DIAGNOSIS

Jack is suffering from AORTIC STENOSIS. His heart murmur is caused by turbulence in the blood passing through a narrowed aortic valve, which was visible on his angiogram. The enlargement of the left ventricle is the result of the extra work it has been doing to force the blood through the narrowed valve.

The cause of Jack's heart valve problem is not known, but his doctor believes that he will soon experience failure of the left side of his heart. He strongly advises that Jack have surgery immediately.

TREATMENT

Jack's aortic valve is replaced with a valve from a pig. The result is a striking improvement in his condition – so great an improvement that Jack realizes, for the first time, how severely disabled he had become.

THE FOLLOW-UP

Six years after his operation, Jack is still playing an active game of tennis and is free of symptoms.

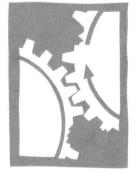

HEART MUSCLE DISEASE

MOST HEART PROBLEMS CAN be traced to high blood pressure, congenital defects, or an underlying disease that affects the blood supply to the heart or the heart valves. However, occasionally, the primary cause of a heart problem is a disease affecting the heart muscle itself, or the tough membrane, known as the pericardium, that surrounds the heart.

The principal disorders of the heart muscle are different forms of cardiomyopathy (which means simply "disease of the heart muscle") and myocarditis (inflammation of the heart muscle). In rare cases, the heart may also be affected by a tumor. The primary disorder affecting the pericardium is an inflammatory condition called pericarditis, which can be caused by viruses, bacteria, autoimmune disorders, and heart attacks.

CARDIOMYOPATHY

Cardiomyopathy may occur as one manifestation of a disease affecting many body organs, such as systemic lupus erythematosus, sarcoidosis, alcoholism, or amyloidosis, or may be caused by poisoning of the heart, infection with bacteria or viruses, a genetic or biochemical disorder, vitamin or mineral

FORMS OF CARDIOMYOPATHY

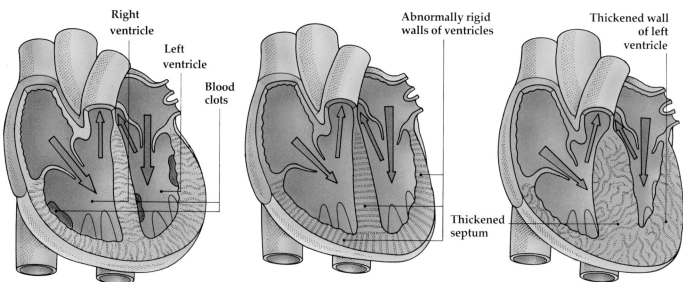

Dilated cardiomyopathy
In this form, there is a ballooning (dilation) of the lower heart chambers (ventricles). They contract less forcefully and eject too little blood with each contraction. This leads to heart failure, a condition in which the heart is unable to maintain the circulation of the blood at a sufficient volume to provide enough oxygen to the tissues. Clots often form on the inner walls of the chambers.

Restrictive cardiomyopathy
In this condition, the walls of the lower heart chambers are abnormally rigid and do not allow for normal filling. This usually occurs because the muscle has been altered by the deposition within it of scar tissue or some other material, such as iron or protein. Symptoms of restrictive cardiomyopathy include swelling of the ankles and fluid accumulation in the abdomen and lungs.

Hypertrophic cardiomyopathy
In this form, portions of the heart muscle become abnormally thickened – especially the wall of the left ventricle and the partition (septum) between the two sides of the heart. The thickening occurs as a result of overgrowth of the constituent muscle fibers. Unlike most cases of heart enlargement, there is no obvious underlying cause in hypertrophic cardiomyopathy.

deficiency, or unknown causes. There are three kinds of cardiomyopathy – dilated, hypertrophic, and restrictive (see FORMS OF CARDIOMYOPATHY, below left). Whatever the type, the end result is eventually heart failure (see page 104).

Dilated cardiomyopathy

This form of cardiomyopathy is most common in middle-aged men. Eventually, heart failure causes symptoms such as severe breathlessness, palpitations, swelling of the ankles, and sometimes vague pain in the chest.

Alcoholic cardiomyopathy

Alcoholic cardiomyopathy is a type of dilated cardiomyopathy. It leads to heart failure, with symptoms similar to those described above.

Overindulgence in alcohol can affect the heart in three ways. First, because some heavy drinkers consume few nutrients other than those in alcohol, they tend to have vitamin deficiencies, which damage the heart. Second, additives in alcoholic drinks can poison the heart. Third, alcohol can have a direct toxic effect on the heart, which commonly occurs in people who consume large quantities (6 to 8 ounces or more a day) of alcohol over a period of many years.

Hypertrophic cardiomyopathy

Many people with hypertrophic cardiomyopathy, in which portions of the heart become abnormally thickened, have no symptoms. The first sign of this disorder may be sudden death, which usually occurs in children or young adults during, or just after, strenuous exertion. When symptoms do occur, the most common are breathlessness, angina, fatigue, and fainting.

At least half of all cases of hypertrophic cardiomyopathy have a genetic (hereditary) cause. The close relatives of people with this condition are commonly found to be affected as well, although they may not have any symptoms.

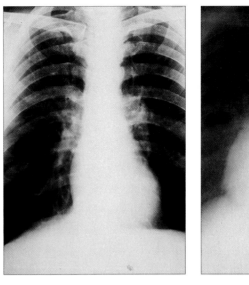

Restrictive cardiomyopathy

In this condition, there is a raised back pressure in the veins because the heart chambers are not able to fill properly. The results are swollen ankles, accumulation of fluid in the abdomen and lungs, and enlargement of the liver.

Treatment

The treatment of cardiomyopathy depends on treating or removing the underlying cause, if one can be found. If heart failure develops, it can be treated with drugs, but, for many patients, the only hope of survival is a heart transplant.

MYOCARDITIS

Myocarditis is an inflammation of the heart muscle that is usually caused by a virus infection. It may also result from other causes, such as rheumatic fever and other autoimmune disorders, drugs, chemicals, and radiation. Myocarditis often remains unsuspected until it shows up during a routine electrocardiogram examination; in other cases, it causes vague chest pain and shortness of breath. For most people, recovery is complete. However, severe cases, especially in young children and pregnant women, may progress to heart rhythm disturbance, heart block, and heart failure, in which case myocarditis may be fatal.

Alcohol and the heart
These chest X-rays show the outline of a normal heart (above left) and the outline of a heart that has become dilated, or enlarged, due to alcohol abuse (above).

If drinking is stopped before heart failure occurs, the progression of the disease may be halted and, in some cases, reversed. However, once heart failure develops from this cause, the outlook is poor; less than 25 percent of alcoholics with heart failure survive for more than 3 years. The only hope for them is abstinence.

PERICARDITIS

Pericarditis is an inflammation of the pericardium, the sac that encloses the heart. The pericardium has two parts, a tough outer bag (the fibrous pericardium) and an inner membrane (the serous pericardium), which has two layers. One layer covers the outside of the heart and the other lines the fibrous pericardium. These two layers are separated by a thin film of lubricating fluid that is secreted by the inner layer.

The most common causes of pericarditis are virus infection and heart attack. Pericarditis may also occur as a complication of another disease such as rheumatic fever, kidney failure, or cancer.

What are its effects?

Pericarditis causes pain behind the breastbone that can be worse in certain positions or when swallowing or breathing deeply. Friction between roughened areas on the two layers of the serous pericardium can cause a pericardial rub, which is audible with a stethoscope and synchronous with the pulse.

Acute inflammation may cause the two layers of the serous pericardium to stick together, thus restricting the free action of the heart. Inflammation may also cause the inner layer to produce more than the normal amount of fluid. This is known as a pericardial effusion and may cause severe compression of the heart (cardiac tamponade). The condition may diminish the ability of the heart to maintain the circulation, which can cause shock.

Constrictive pericarditis is a chronic condition that causes a slow, progressive tightening of the pericardium as a result of scar tissue. This has a severe effect on the ability of the heart to fill with blood between contractions, which causes a damming of blood in the veins and enlargement of the liver. As a result, fluid collects in the abdomen and sometimes elsewhere in the body.

Constrictive pericarditis is readily remedied by the surgical removal of the thickened, inelastic pericardium.

HEART TUMORS

All heart tumors are rare. Most are secondary tumors (cancers that have spread from other parts of the body).

Primary tumors (arising from the heart itself) are usually benign. The most common primary tumors are myxomas – soft, gelatinous masses about 1 to 3 inches in diameter. They are connected by a stalk to the wall of one of the upper heart chambers (atria). The sound of the tumor striking the wall of the heart chamber can often be heard by a doctor through a stethoscope. A myxoma can be removed by open heart surgery.

THE STRUCTURE OF THE PERICARDIUM

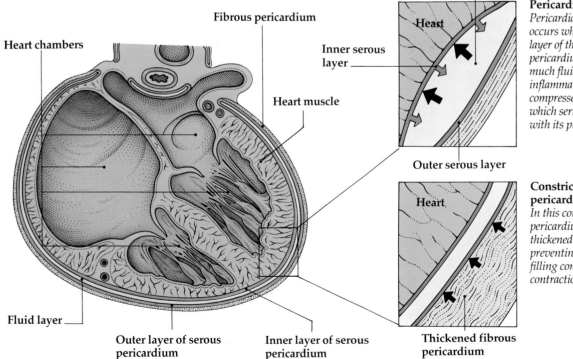

Heart chambers

Fibrous pericardium

Inner serous layer

Heart muscle

Fluid layer

Outer layer of serous pericardium

Inner layer of serous pericardium

Fluid collection

Heart

Outer serous layer

Thickened fibrous pericardium

Pericardial effusion
Pericardial effusion occurs when the inner layer of the serous pericardium produces too much fluid as a result of inflammation. The fluid compresses the heart, which seriously interferes with its pumping action.

Constrictive pericarditis
In this condition, the pericardium becomes thickened and inelastic, preventing the heart from filling completely between contractions.

CASE HISTORY
CHEST PAIN AND PALPITATIONS

L AWRENCE IS A BIG MAN in every respect – in body, personality, energy, and ideas. All his life he has been an energetic worker and an enthusiastic sportsman. However, recently, Lawrence's wife was alarmed by his accounts of a thumping sensation in his chest, chest pains, and feeling faint. She insisted he see his doctor.

PERSONAL DETAILS
Name Lawrence Littleton
Age 53
Occupation Police chief
Family Lawrence's father, grandfather, and a younger brother died suddenly from a heart disorder while apparently in good health.

THE CONSULTATION
The doctor's questions establish that Lawrence's chest pain is angina. Examination shows that Lawrence's heart is considerably enlarged and an ECG shows frequent premature beats – the cause of the thumping in Lawrence's chest. His doctor refers him to a cardiologist.

THE SPECIALIST CONSULTATION
The cardiologist orders an echocardiogram, which shows that Lawrence's heart is greatly enlarged due to thickening of the wall of the left ventricle (lower pumping chamber) and of the wall separating the two sides of the heart.

Examining the chest
When the doctor feels the left side of Lawrence's chest, he detects an unusually powerful heartbeat – a clue to Lawrence's problem, which is an overgrown heart muscle.

The cardiologist then performs special tests involving injections of dye to measure the output of blood from Lawrence's heart. The tests reveal that the output is reduced at rest and does not increase normally with exercise. This is why Lawrence has been feeling faint when he exerts himself. After discussion with the cardiologist, Lawrence agrees to an unusual procedure in which a tiny sample of heart muscle is taken (biopsied) from the inside of his heart by means of a cardiac catheter.

THE DIAGNOSIS
Examination of the sample confirms that the enlargement is caused by thickening of the heart muscle fibers, which are arranged in a disorganized manner.

The findings add up to a diagnosis of HYPERTROPHIC CARDIOMYOPATHY, an inherited disorder. Evidence of the condition is frequently found in a sufferer's immediate relatives, who appear to be free of symptoms but who often die suddenly.

Although the coronary arteries supplying blood to Lawrence's heart are normal, the amount of tissue they must supply is greatly increased, so the heart muscle is not getting enough blood. This is the reason for Lawrence's angina. The main problem in hypertrophic cardiomyopathy is a reduction in the volume of blood pumped with each beat. In severe cases, the output is so low that heart failure results.

THE TREATMENT
Left-sided heart failure has already developed. A few months later Lawrence experiences severe failure of both sides of his heart. He is told that his only hope for survival is a heart transplant. Lawrence agrees to the operation and is now waiting for a suitable donor.

SURGICAL PROCEDURES
HEART TRANSPLANTATION

HEART TRANSPLANTATION **is generally reserved for people under 55 who have terminal heart failure. It offers a last hope of survival after other medical and surgical treatments have been unsuccessfully attempted. About 80 percent of people who receive a heart transplant today survive for 5 years, but the procedure is not without serious risks.**

Most candidates for heart transplantation have suffered a widespread loss of functioning heart muscle, either from repeated heart attacks or from cardiomyopathy. People who have any other active diseases, such as severe diabetes, liver or kidney disorders, cancer, or major infections, are usually not suitable for a transplant. Patients with certain lung diseases may be better suited for a heart-lung transplant rather than a heart transplant alone.

Criteria for transplantation

For a transplant to be performed, a suitable donor heart must be available. In addition, the donor's relatives must give consent for the heart to be used for transplantation. The blood group of the donor must be the same as that of the recipient, and other characteristics of the donor's and recipient's tissues – known as their tissue types – must match as closely as possible.

Few donors are available, so relatively few people who are suitable for a heart transplant can actually be given one. Receiving a transplant depends largely on the good fortune of a suitable donor heart being available at the right place and at the right time.

Risks

To prevent rejection of the donor heart by the recipient's immune system (which is fatal unless a second transplant can be performed), immunosuppressant drugs are given. Even with drugs, the donor heart is sometimes rejected; if rejection occurs, it usually happens within the first 6 weeks after surgery. Immunosuppression itself can also have life-threatening complications, including the risk of overwhelming infection.

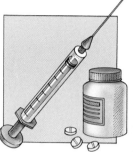

1 To reduce the chances of rejection of the transplanted heart by the recipient's immune system, immunosuppressant drugs (left) are given to inhibit the immune system. Treatment with immunosuppressant drugs is started before the operation and must be continued for the rest of the patient's life.

Site of incision

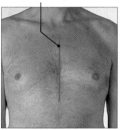

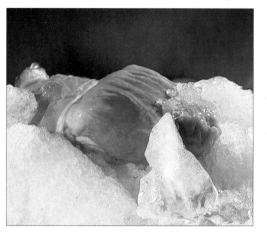

2 The donor heart is obtained from someone who has recently been pronounced brain dead, usually after an accident, but whose heart is healthy and is being kept functioning by artificial means. After removal from the donor, the heart and coronary arteries are washed and flushed out with a maintenance fluid. The heart is then packed in ice (above), where it can be preserved for several hours before it is inserted into the recipient.

3 An incision is made in the recipient's breastbone, which is split apart, and the pericardium (sac covering the heart) is cut to gain access to the heart.

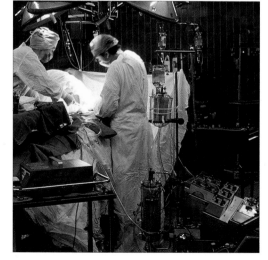

4 The patient is connected to a heart-lung machine (left), which takes over the function of the heart and lungs. Deoxygenated blood is removed from the patient via cannulas inserted into the venae cavae, oxygenated in the heart-lung machine, and then returned to the patient via a cannula inserted into the aorta.

5 The diseased heart is stopped by clamping the aorta; most of the heart is then removed by cutting through the walls of the upper heart chambers (atria) and the arteries to the lungs (pulmonary artery) and body (aorta). The back walls of the atria are left in place (right).

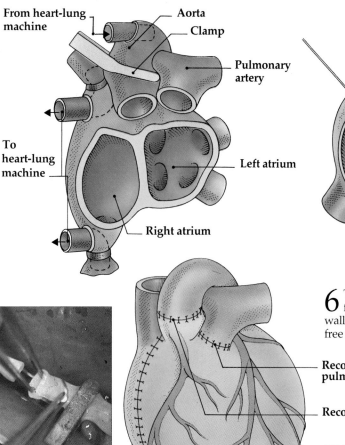

From heart-lung machine

Aorta

Clamp

Pulmonary artery

To heart-lung machine

Left atrium

Right atrium

Donor heart

6 The donor heart is stitched to the free edge of the left atrium, the wall between the two atria, and the free edge of the right atrium (above).

Reconnection to pulmonary artery

Reconnection to aorta

7 To complete the main part of the operation, the patient's pulmonary artery and aorta are connected to the donor heart (left).

8 Smaller blood vessels are reconnected (above). The surgeon then removes air from the heart chambers and removes the clamp on the aorta to restore a blood supply to the heart muscle. The heart is then started, usually by warming it; if this doesn't work, the heart is started by applying an electric shock (right).

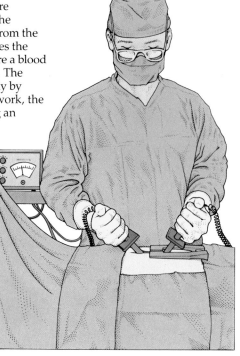

9 Finally, the surgeon checks for and repairs any small leaks from blood vessels, disconnects the patient from the heart-lung machine, and closes the chest.

AFTER THE OPERATION

Following a transplant operation, the patient is taken to the surgical cardiac intensive-care unit and his or her condition is monitored for any signs of rejection of the new heart or for signs of infection. Immediately after the operation, the patient is connected to a ventilator to assist breathing and is under continuous electrocardiographic monitoring. Several drainage tubes are also placed inside the chest. These are removed or disconnected as recovery proceeds. After being discharged from the hospital, the patient usually returns for heart muscle biopsies to check for any signs of heart tissue rejection. Most forms of physical activity can be gradually resumed under a doctor's directions.

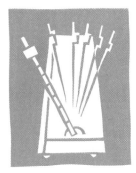

HEART RATE AND RHYTHM DISORDERS

THE HEALTHY HEART BEATS regularly at a rate of 60 to 100 beats per minute during rest. It is normal for this rate to speed up during any form of exercise or in response to stress. However, in general, if you feel your heart beating irregularly or at an abnormally fast or slow rate (conditions known as arrhythmias), some form of treatment may be required to restore a normal rhythm and rate.

The treatment of arrhythmias has progressed rapidly in recent years. Many new drugs have been developed to control these heart disorders safely and effectively. There have also been advances in the design of pacemakers and defibrillators, devices that can correct the heart's rhythm and speed.

TYPES OF ARRHYTHMIAS

There are two types of arrhythmias – the tachycardias, in which the heart rate is faster than 100 beats per minute, and the bradycardias, in which the rate falls below 60 beats per minute. These groups are classified further according to rhythm and according to whether the electrical impulses that trigger each heartbeat originate in the sinoatrial node (specialized cells at the top of the heart) or in another part of the heart.

If there is a fault in the conducting system of the heart, the pattern of beats may also vary. Instead of each beat of the atria being followed by a beat of the ventricles, there may be multiple beats of the atria for each beat of the ventricles or the ventricles may beat completely independently of the atria.

What causes an arrhythmia?

The most common cause of an arrhythmia is coronary heart disease, narrowing or blockage of the arteries that supply the heart. As a result of an inadequate blood

WHAT ARE THE SYMPTOMS OF AN ARRHYTHMIA?

If a tachycardia starts suddenly, it may cause palpitations, a fluttering sensation in the chest. But many people who think they have palpitations actually have a normal heartbeat. They have simply become more aware of it.

Both tachycardias and bradycardias can cause dizziness or sudden fainting by reducing the efficiency of the heart. This reduced efficiency diminishes the flow of blood to the brain. In addition, tachycardias and bradycardias can also cause breathlessness, because a heart that is beating less efficiently pumps less blood through the lungs.

NORMAL AND ABNORMAL HEARTBEATS

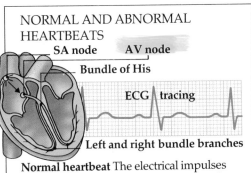

Normal heartbeat The electrical impulses that trigger each heartbeat originate in the sinoatrial (SA) node, the heart's pacemaker. The impulses spread through the upper chambers to the atrioventricular (AV) node. Then the current slows before traveling along conducting muscle fibers – the bundle of His and its two branches – to the lower chambers.

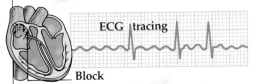

Atrial fibrillation Impulses follow a circular route in the atria, making them beat at a rate of 250 to 350 beats per minute. Blockage at the AV node prevents the ventricles from picking up all the impulses from the atria and they beat erratically.

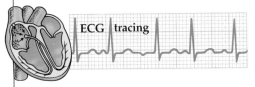

Multifocal atrial tachycardia Impulses originate irregularly and at different points in the atria. The rate is more than 100 beats per minute.

supply, the specialized cells that produce and transmit electrical impulses through the heart stop working properly. The damage may develop over several months or suddenly after a heart attack. In people with coronary heart disease, the heart becomes more irritable, so that minor stresses such as smoking or coffee cause an arrhythmia.

Arrhythmias in rare cases may be caused by a congenital abnormality in part of the heart's electrical conducting system. Although the abnormality is present from birth, it often causes the arrhythmia only later in life. Strenuous exercise, any chemical disturbance, certain drugs, and substances such as coffee may trigger this type of arrhythmia.

Because the hormones produced by the thyroid gland act as a stimulant on the heart, any type of thyroid disorder may affect the heartbeat. A persistent tachycardia may be due to an abnormally active thyroid gland, while a bradycardia may result from an underactive thyroid gland. Thyroid disorders may also trigger atrial flutter or fibrillation (a more disorganized version of flutter).

How is an arrhythmia diagnosed?

If your doctor suspects that you have an abnormal heartbeat, he or she will first listen to your chest through a stethoscope to assess your heart's rate and rhythm. Your pulse will also be taken to help evaluate how efficiently your heart is pumping blood.

The exact type of arrhythmia may be established by electrocardiography (see page 50), which shows the rate and pattern of electrical activity in the heart. If the arrhythmia occurs intermittently, it is usually necessary to make a continuous 24-hour recording using a portable ECG machine called a Holter monitor.

The doctor may also take a blood sample to test for thyroid overactivity or any other chemical imbalance that may be causing the problem.

TAKING THE PULSE

The pulse is the rhythmic movement of the muscular wall of an artery as blood is pumped through it. A doctor assesses the pulse in an artery by pressing one or more fingers against the skin covering it. The rate, rhythm, strength, and character of the pulse, and whether the artery feels soft or hard, provide important clues to the nature of any heart or circulatory disorder that is present.

Because the pulse rate usually corresponds to the heart rate, it is a useful measure of how regularly fast or slow the heart is working. Occasionally, however, when the heart is beating very rapidly, some of the beats may be too weak to expand the artery wall, causing the pulse to be slower than the actual heart rate.

Neck

Front of elbow

Groin

Back of knee

Front of wrist

Foot

Where is the pulse taken?
The pulse is usually taken at the wrist, just below the base of the thumb. However, it may also be felt in the neck, at the front of the elbow, in the groin, behind the knee, and in two places on the foot.

Water-hammer pulse
If the artery wall expands greatly and collapses quickly (the so-called water-hammer pulse), the aortic valve may be failing to close properly. This pulse (below) is best felt at the wrist with the person's arm raised.

Normal pulse

Character of pulse
The character or shape of the pulse, best felt in the neck, provides important clues to the diagnosis.

Slow rising pulse
An artery wall that expands only a little and slowly may be caused by narrowing of the aortic valve (aortic stenosis).

Alternating high and low pulse
This suggests serious heart failure, with the left ventricle struggling to keep up with its work load.

TREATING ARRHYTHMIAS

Many different drugs are used to treat arrhythmias. Most act by slowing down the transmission of nerve impulses in the heart muscle, thus producing a calming effect on the heart. These antiarrhythmic drugs include beta blockers (see page 129), calcium channel blockers (see page 132), cardiac glycosides such as digitalis (see page 128), and specific antiarrhythmic drugs such as lidocaine, quinidine, and procainamide. The type of drug chosen depends on the type of arrhythmia, although several different drugs may be suitable for a particular condition. Drug treatment may not completely restore the heartbeat to normal, but, by improving the pumping efficiency of the heart, treatment can relieve symptoms.

Doctors also treat arrhythmias by inserting a pacemaker into the body or by passing an electric shock through the heart (defibrillation).

PACING THE HEART

Every year tens of thousands of Americans have a pacemaker implanted because the heart has started to beat too slowly or erratically to keep the body supplied with enough blood.

Pacemaker
A pacemaker consists of a battery-powered pulse generator and an electrical wire that is attached to the heart. Modern pacemakers are about the size of a sandwich cookie and weigh between 2 and 4 ounces.

Electrical wire to heart

Pulse generator

INSERTION OF PACEMAKER

Inserting a pacemaker is a simple procedure. In most cases, the electrical wire is passed through a neck vein and guided down into the heart. It can also be introduced through the front of the chest and attached to the outside of the heart. The power source is then fitted under a flap of skin either below the collarbone or in the abdomen.

A local anesthetic is injected to deaden the tissues in the areas where the wire and power source will be inserted. The procedure usually takes less than half an hour and recovery is rapid. Complications are rare and normal activities can usually be resumed after one day in the hospital, although strenuous exercise should be avoided for 2 weeks.

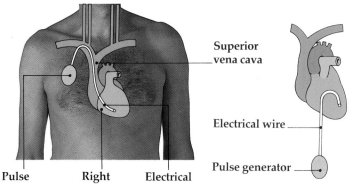

Superior vena cava

Electrical wire

Pulse generator

Pulse generator **Right ventricle** **Electrical wire**

Transvenous implantation
As shown above, the wire is introduced into a vein at the shoulder or the base of the neck. One end is guided into the heart chamber. The power source is attached to the free end and implanted into a pocket created between the skin and muscle of the chest.

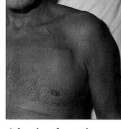

After implantation
Once the pacemaker is in place, it appears as a small lump under the skin.

Epicardial implantation
If the patient is undergoing heart surgery, a pacemaker can be fitted at the same time. As shown above, the electrical wire is attached to the outside of the heart muscle (the epicardium) and the power source is implanted under the skin of the abdomen.

X-ray of pacemaker
This X-ray shows a pacemaker in the chest. The electronic circuitry is visible in the top half of the generator. Lithium batteries are located in the lower section. The wire sutures down the center of the chest indicate that the person has had a previous heart operation.

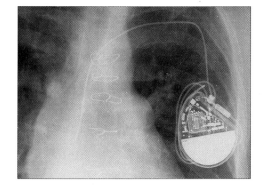

Types of pacemakers

A pacemaker is a small, battery-operated device that sends timed electrical impulses to the heart to make it contract and keep it beating at a regular rate.

Several different types of pacemakers are available. Some supply electrical impulses at a fixed rate, which override any activity that the heart is still able to generate. Others work on a demand basis so that the pacemaker turns off when the heart beats normally; when the heart slows down or misses a beat, the pacemaker starts again. Programmable pacemakers can be adjusted to work either at a fixed rate or on demand. They can also be programmed to work at a faster or slower rate to suit the patient's needs.

Pacemakers usually run for several years before the lithium battery runs down. Periodic checkups ensure that the instrument is still working properly. When the batteries need to be replaced, a minor operation with the use of a local anesthetic is performed to open the skin flap and replace the power source.

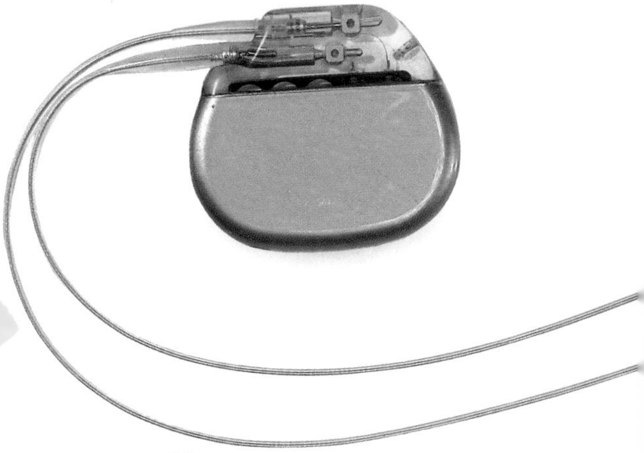

Dual-chamber pacemakers
Some advanced pacemakers, such as the one shown at right, have two electrical wires. One is positioned in the atria to start them contracting properly, the other is positioned in the ventricles. These dual-chamber pacemakers improve the filling of the ventricles; the pacemaker's output responds automatically to changes in the person's activities, adjusting the rate as required.
The illustration shows the position of the pacemaker wires in the heart chambers.

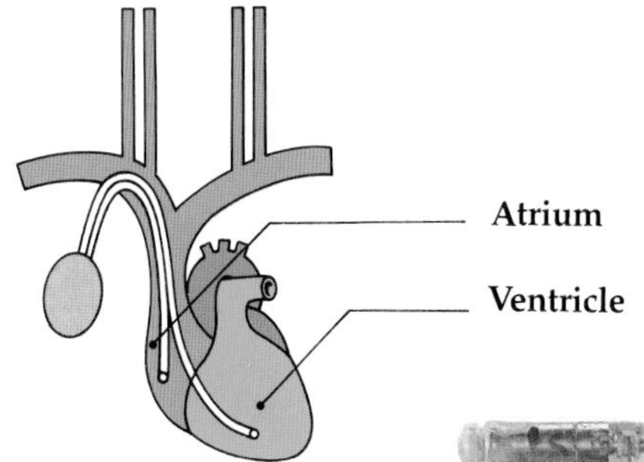

Atrium

Ventricle

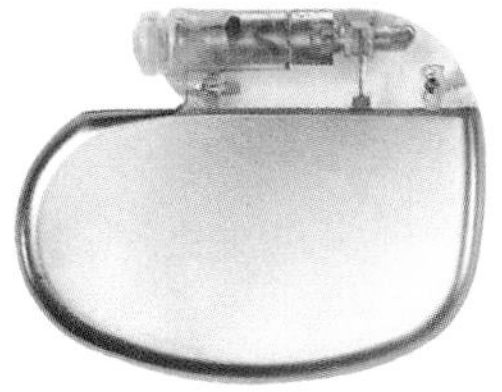

Programmable pacemaker
This type of pacemaker can be programmed to work at a fixed rate or on demand; the rate of discharge is also adjustable. The pacemaker is programmed by sending electromagnetic signals through the skin from an external device.

HEART REGULATOR

A recently developed device called the automatic implantable cardiac defibrillator can, like other types of defibrillators (see page 103), return a rapidly beating heart to a normal speed and rhythm. This defibrillator is considered only after all other medical measures have failed.

The automatic implantable cardiac defibrillator is useful in the treatment of patients who have repeated episodes of ventricular tachycardia (rapid heartbeats). People who have this device may survive an otherwise fatal arrhythmia. The device consists of a small electric generator with three wires. The generator is implanted in a pocket created under the abdominal skin. One wire is inserted through an incision in the left side of the chest and is attached to the lower surface of the heart. The other two wires are inserted into a neck vein; one is fed into the right atrium, the other is positioned in the right ventricle.

When the automatic implantable cardiac defibrillator detects a speeding up of the heartbeat, it administers an electric shock. The burst of electricity stops the heart from beating for a split second, allowing the sinoatrial node to regain control of the heart's rhythm. The defibrillator discharges again if the arrhythmia continues, up to a maximum of four times. When the device discharges, it feels like a blow to the chest. Patients learn to anticipate it by recognizing the symptoms of tachycardia, which include sudden faintness and breathlessness.

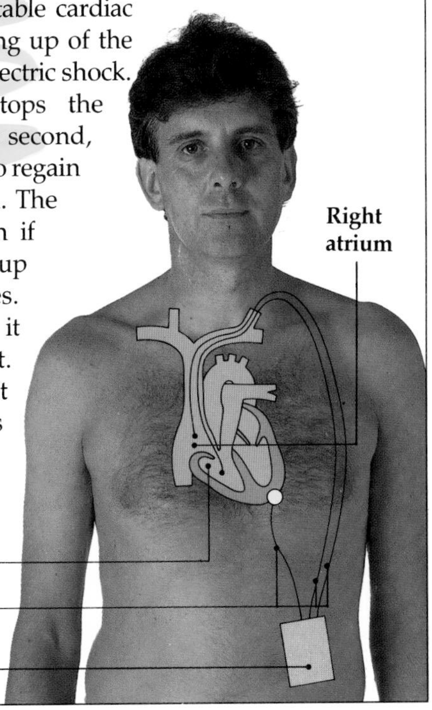

Right atrium

Right ventricle

Electrical wires

Generator

MONITOR YOUR SYMPTOMS
PALPITATIONS

Palpitations (irregular or unusually fast or strong heart-beats) normally occur after strenuous exercise because the heart has been working harder. However, if you have palpitations that occur for no obvious reason, consult your doctor, especially if the palpitations recur over several days or are accompanied by pain or breathlessness.

> **WARNING**
> In some people, anxiety can result in panic attacks – feelings of extreme fear with symptoms such as palpitations, breathlessness, and sweating. If you have any doubt about the cause of such symptoms, call your doctor immediately.

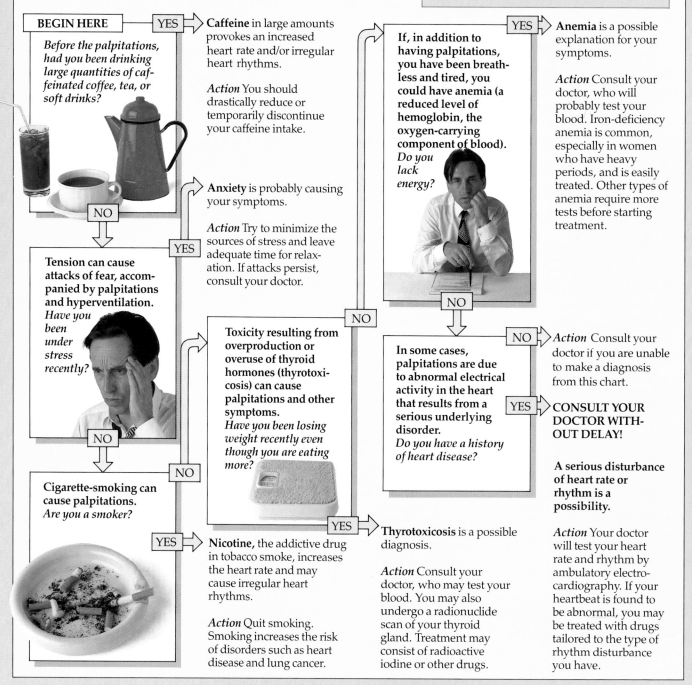

BEGIN HERE — YES ▷

Before the palpitations, had you been drinking large quantities of caffeinated coffee, tea, or soft drinks?

Caffeine in large amounts provokes an increased heart rate and/or irregular heart rhythms.

Action You should drastically reduce or temporarily discontinue your caffeine intake.

NO

Tension can cause attacks of fear, accompanied by palpitations and hyperventilation. *Have you been under stress recently?*

YES ▷ **Anxiety** is probably causing your symptoms.

Action Try to minimize the sources of stress and leave adequate time for relaxation. If attacks persist, consult your doctor.

NO

Cigarette-smoking can cause palpitations. *Are you a smoker?*

NO ▷ **Toxicity resulting from overproduction or overuse of thyroid hormones (thyrotoxicosis) can cause palpitations and other symptoms.** *Have you been losing weight recently even though you are eating more?*

YES ▷ **Nicotine,** the addictive drug in tobacco smoke, increases the heart rate and may cause irregular heart rhythms.

Action Quit smoking. Smoking increases the risk of disorders such as heart disease and lung cancer.

YES ▷ **Thyrotoxicosis** is a possible diagnosis.

Action Consult your doctor, who may test your blood. You may also undergo a radionuclide scan of your thyroid gland. Treatment may consist of radioactive iodine or other drugs.

If, in addition to having palpitations, you have been breathless and tired, you could have anemia (a reduced level of hemoglobin, the oxygen-carrying component of blood). *Do you lack energy?*

YES ▷ **Anemia** is a possible explanation for your symptoms.

Action Consult your doctor, who will probably test your blood. Iron-deficiency anemia is common, especially in women who have heavy periods, and is easily treated. Other types of anemia require more tests before starting treatment.

NO

In some cases, palpitations are due to abnormal electrical activity in the heart that results from a serious underlying disorder. *Do you have a history of heart disease?*

NO ▷ *Action* Consult your doctor if you are unable to make a diagnosis from this chart.

YES ▷ **CONSULT YOUR DOCTOR WITH-OUT DELAY!**

A serious disturbance of heart rate or rhythm is a possibility.

Action Your doctor will test your heart rate and rhythm by ambulatory electro-cardiography. If your heartbeat is found to be abnormal, you may be treated with drugs tailored to the type of rhythm disturbance you have.

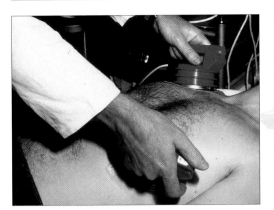

Defibrillator
A defibrillator consists of a machine that produces an electric current and two metal plates that are placed on the patient's chest. The machine also incorporates ECG leads so that the person's heart rate and rhythm can be continuously monitored.

How external defibrillation is performed

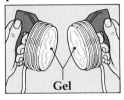

Gel

1 Conducting gel or paste is first applied evenly to the metal plates.

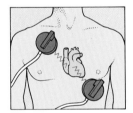

2 The plates are pressed firmly against the chest and a burst of electricity is sent through the heart.

HOW DOES DEFIBRILLATION WORK?

Defibrillation works by stopping the heart from beating for a split second and allowing the sinoatrial node to regain control over the electrical impulses passing through the heart. More than one burst of electricity is often needed before the heart starts beating normally.

GIVING THE HEART A SHOCK

Sudden rapid or uncoordinated beating of the heart can be treated by passing a brief electric current through the heart. The technique, called defibrillation or cardioversion, may be performed in two ways. In external defibrillation, two metal plates are placed on the front of the chest. In internal defibrillation, sometimes used during heart surgery, the plates are held in contact with the heart.

External defibrillation is used to treat the sudden onset of certain types of arrhythmia, usually tachycardia (abnormally rapid heartbeat) or fibrillation (rapid, uncoordinated heartbeat from either the atria or the ventricles). It is usually needed when a severe arrhythmia develops just after a heart attack.

Occasionally a drug, such as lidocaine (a type of anesthetic), is injected into the circulation before the procedure to help stabilize the activity inside the heart muscle. If defibrillation is done in an emergency when someone has collapsed, no painkillers or sedatives are needed. However, if defibrillation is being performed as a planned treatment in someone who has had an arrhythmia for several hours and is fully conscious, a preliminary medication is usually given.

The people giving the treatment must not touch the patient or the bed when the defibrillator is activated, because the electric shock could interfere with the function of their hearts.

ASK YOUR DOCTOR
HEART RATE AND RHYTHM DISORDERS

Q My uncle died suddenly a month ago, and the autopsy showed that he had suffered a massive heart attack. Could a defibrillator have saved his life?

A Many people who have a heart attack die despite having a defibrillator used on them. Sometimes the heart is so badly damaged it just stops beating and nothing can get it going again. In other cases, an arrhythmia triggered by the heart attack refuses to respond to either drug treatment or electric shocks.

Q My heart occasionally feels as though it is missing a beat, so my doctor arranged for me to have a 24-hour ECG. I have been reassured that the tracing showed only an occasional irregular beat, but shouldn't my heart beat regularly the whole time?

A No one has a heart that beats perfectly. A few irregular beats can occur in normal hearts and are nothing to worry about.

Q Every time I play tennis I suffer from palpitations for about an hour afterward. Is there something wrong with my heart?

A Strenuous exercise is supposed to increase the speed of your heartbeat, and when the heart beats more rapidly it can cause palpitations in some people. However, once you rest, your heart rate should quickly return to normal. Anyone who suffers palpitations after exercise that last longer than a few minutes needs a checkup. Your doctor will probably give you an exercise ECG to see if exertion triggers an arrhythmia.

HEART FAILURE

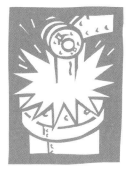

T HE POPULAR IDEA THAT HEART FAILURE means failure of the heart to continue to beat is wrong. Heart failure means that the heart cannot keep up with the task of pumping blood to the lungs and body tissues. The condition is often serious, but it does not mean that the heart has stopped or is about to stop, or that the person who has heart failure is in imminent danger of dying.

Heart failure affects about one person in 100. The degree of failure varies. In some people it may be so small that doctors are unable to determine easily whether it is present or not; in others it may produce severe symptoms. Treatment can prolong a life, but about 45 percent of men and 30 percent of women with persistent heart failure die within 3 years.

CAUSES AND SYMPTOMS

The most common causes of heart failure are inadequate blood supply to the heart from coronary artery disease, and continued strain on the heart from long-

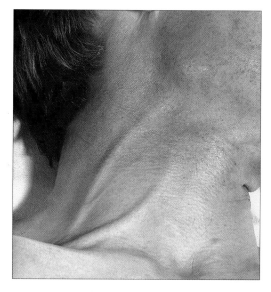

Raised venous pressure
The increased pressure in the veins, due to heart failure, is clearly visible in the prominent jugular veins of the patient shown above.

standing high blood pressure. Other causes include heart valve disease, diabetes, anemia, direct damage to the heart muscle from drugs, alcohol or other toxic agents, lung disease, pericarditis, and vitamin B_1 deficiency.

Heart failure can occur when a normal heart is called on to beat fast or hard all the time. This problem sometimes develops in conditions such as thyroid gland overactivity, in which the body's metabolic rate is greatly increased; anemia, in which the blood must circulate more rapidly to carry the same amount of oxygen; and high blood pressure, in which the heart must pump harder against increased resistance. Correction of the underlying cause of the rapid beat usually relieves the heart failure.

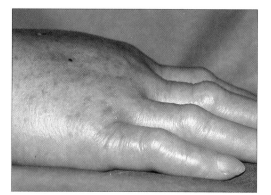

Severe edema
At first, edema may cause only a slight weight gain and swelling of the ankles. Once the fluid in the body increases by more than about 15 percent, swelling may become apparent in many parts of the body, including the hands.

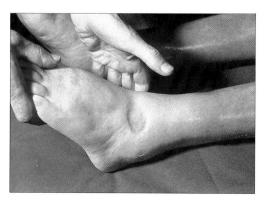

Peripheral edema
Firmly pressing a finger into an area of skin affected by edema displaces fluid and leaves a visible indentation. The movement of fluid through the walls of the capillaries is very slow and it may take up to 20 minutes before the depression disappears.

HOW HEART FAILURE AFFECTS THE CIRCULATION

In heart failure, the heart has a reduced pumping capacity. As a result, blood collects in the veins, creating a backward pressure that forces fluid into the surrounding tissues. The effect on the body varies according to whether the left or right side of the heart is involved, as illustrated below.

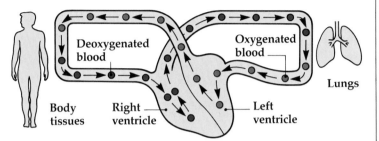

Body tissues · **Right ventricle** · Deoxygenated blood · Oxygenated blood · **Left ventricle** · **Lungs**

Normal circulation
When the heart is working normally, the two sides of the heart pump out the same amount of blood with each beat, and each side takes in the same amount as it pumps out. This means that there is no buildup or congestion of blood anywhere in the circulation.

Right-sided heart failure | **Left-sided heart failure**

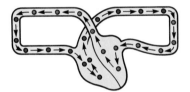
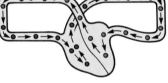

1 The right side of the heart cannot pump out blood (circles) as fast as it returns from the body via the veins.

1 The left side of the heart cannot pump out blood (circles) as fast as it returns from the lungs via the veins.

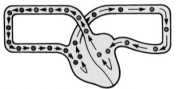

2 Gradually, the veins become congested with blood.

2 The lungs become congested with blood.

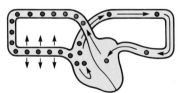
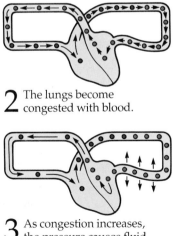

3 As the congestion increases, the pressure forces fluid into the surrounding tissues, causing them to swell.

3 As congestion increases, the pressure causes fluid to collect in the lungs. This displaces air from the air sacs, causing breathlessness.

The effect on the body

Heart failure can affect the right side of the heart, the left side of the heart, or both. Failure of the left side causes back pressure in the blood vessels of the lungs, thus reducing the transfer of oxygen from the air to the blood. Fluid collects in the lungs, reducing the surface area in the lungs available for transfer of oxygen to the blood. Breathlessness (the main symptom of heart failure of the left side of the heart), cough, fatigue, and blueness of the skin may result.

Failure of the right side of the heart causes increased back pressure in the veins draining blood from the rest of the body. Fluid then collects in the tissues, causing swelling (edema) in the ankles and lower back, distention of the abdomen, and enlargement of the liver. The reduced supply of refreshed blood to the muscles also causes tiredness.

TREATING THE PROBLEM

Drug treatment can control the symptoms (see DRUGS FOR HEART FAILURE on page 127). Diuretics (see page 134) help prevent the buildup of excess fluid in the body because they reduce the amount of fluid reabsorbed by the kidneys and thus increase the output of urine.

The power of the heart muscle can be improved by treatment with digitalis, the active ingredient in cardiac glycoside drugs (see page 128). Digitalis strengthens the contraction of the heart muscle and slows the excessively fast heart rate that occurs as the heart tries to compensate for its poor performance. Vasodilators, drugs that widen blood vessels, can be useful in reducing the load on the heart. The strain on the heart can be reduced further by losing excess weight.

Heart failure caused by thyrotoxicosis, anemia, and high blood pressure can often be reversed if the underlying condition is treated promptly. Failure due to heart valve disease may be corrected by a valve replacement operation.

CASE HISTORY
BREATHLESSNESS

SEVERAL MONTHS AGO, **Beverly had to turn down a small part in a TV commercial that involved rushing up a flight of stairs because, during rehearsal, she became so breathless that she could not continue. Although she has always been slim, close-fitting clothes are becoming uncomfortable and she is having trouble putting on her shoes. Also, for the first time in her life, she has been having palpitations. After waking up one night feeling extremely breathless, she decided to consult her doctor.**

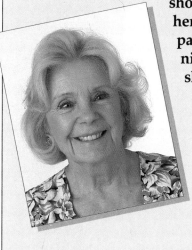

PERSONAL DETAILS
Name Beverly DeSica
Age 60
Occupation Actress
Family No history of significant disease.

THE CONSULTATION
The doctor questions Beverly and then orders a chest X-ray. It shows that both the lower chambers of Beverly's heart are enlarged; the lower parts of the lungs show a haziness caused by fluid collection. The veins in her neck are prominent and appear to pulsate when she sits upright. Her electrocardiogram seems normal but there are occasional premature beats, followed by longer-than-normal pauses. This explains Beverly's palpitations.

Beverly's ankles are obviously swollen. When the doctor presses the swelling, a deep indentation persists for 15 minutes. The doctor tells Beverly that she has heart failure and Beverly is referred to a cardiologist.

Clues to the diagnosis
Beverly's increasing difficulty with putting on her shoes, as a result of edema (fluid collection) affecting her feet and ankles, provides evidence that her heart is failing to keep up with its work load. The heart problem proves to be linked to Beverly's drinking habits.

THE SPECIALIST CONSULTATION
When he listens carefully to Beverly's heart, the cardiologist can find no indication of heart valve disease. However, an echocardiogram reveals that Beverly's heart chambers, especially her left ventricle, are dilated (ballooned out).

Special tests reveal that the amount of blood pumped by Beverly's heart is normal at rest but does not increase with exertion. These findings indicate that Beverly's heart failure is due to cardiomyopathy (a disease of the heart muscle), but they do not demonstrate the underlying cause. When Beverly is questioned about her life-style, she admits that she drinks alcohol every day. Eventually, it becomes clear that she has been consuming more than 12 ounces of hard liquor every day for more than 20 years.

The specialist decides to take a biopsy of muscle from Beverly's heart to confirm the diagnosis.

THE DIAGNOSIS
When the sample is examined, the diagnosis of ALCOHOLIC CARDIO-MYOPATHY is confirmed. The sample shows that some of the muscle fibers have been replaced with scar tissue. This has weakened the power of contraction of Beverly's heart and has led to heart failure.

THE TREATMENT
The doctor tells Beverly that she must stop drinking and refers her to a support group in town. Diuretic drugs help relieve her breathlessness and the edema in the lower part of her body. Small doses of digoxin also improve her condition by strengthening the heart's contractions. After quitting her alcohol habit, she has a reasonable prospect of living for many years.

MECHANICAL AIDS

In certain circumstances, specialized pumping mechanisms can be installed in the body to assist a failing heart in its work of circulating blood around the body. Contrary to optimistic media reports, devices of this kind have not solved the long-term problem of control or correction of heart failure. Today, practical difficulties prohibit these mechanisms from remaining in service for longer than, at most, a few days.

THE INTRA-AORTIC BALLOON PUMP

Intra-aortic balloon pumping is used when a failing heart is expected to recover within a few days, such as after an operation in which the heart is temporarily unable to maintain the circulation.

How is it done?
A long, sausage-shaped balloon is inserted into the aorta. The balloon is electronically timed to inflate between contractions of the left ventricle, which pumps blood into the aorta. Each inflation forces additional blood away from the heart during the periods when the aortic valve is closed. When the left ventricle contracts, the balloon deflates to allow the blood to pass.

Are there any problems?
To place the balloon in the chest, a catheter must be inserted along an artery. This artery remains largely blocked by the balloon's inflation tube, restricting the blood supply to the area that the artery serves. The deprived tissue can suffer severe damage within a few days.

During contractions — Aorta

Aortic valve is open

Balloon deflates

Left ventricle contracts

Coronary arteries receive some blood

Between contractions — Aorta

Aortic valve is closed

Balloon inflates

Left ventricle relaxes

Coronary arteries receive more blood

BYPASS OF THE LEFT SIDE OF THE HEART

Poor circulation due to a failing heart may be improved by using a small pump to perform the function of the main pumping chamber, the left ventricle.

How is it done?
A cannula (connecting tube) is inserted into the vena cava and guided into the left atrium. Oxygenated blood passes down the cannula and into a pump, where it is returned to a femoral artery and up into the aorta.

Are there any problems?
Pumping can be continued for only a short time because the connections in the heart quickly cease to be "watertight." The pump also destroys some of the platelets in the blood, triggering the clotting mechanism.

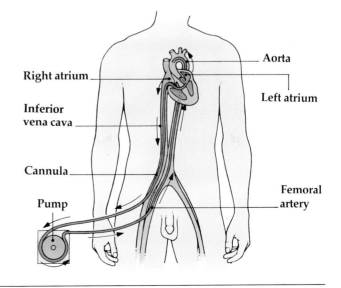

Right atrium

Inferior vena cava

Cannula

Pump

Aorta

Left atrium

Femoral artery

THE ARTIFICIAL HEART

No attempt to reproduce the function of the entire heart has had long-term success. Perhaps the greatest problem is blood clotting. The lining of the natural blood vessels has properties that prevent clotting; it has proved impossible to reproduce those qualities in artificial materials. Artificial hearts have produced large numbers of blood clots that have passed into the circulation. All the patients who have received an artificial heart have died, mostly from strokes, kidney failure, internal bleeding, and infection.

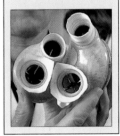

CHAPTER SIX

CIRCULATORY DISEASES

I N PREVIOUS CHAPTERS we have looked at atherosclerosis and how it contributes to heart disease. It is now clear that many people in developed countries greatly increase their risk of coronary heart disease by following a self-indulgent, sedentary life-style. But atherosclerosis is not limited to the coronary arteries; the narrowing process can have serious consequences for every blood vessel in the body.

The heart acts as a pumping station in the circulatory system, which conducts blood (the carrier of vital oxygen and nutrients) to the body's tissues. Just as the pipes of your sink work best when they are unobstructed, so the arteries and veins of your body's circulatory system must be unclogged to be healthy. This chapter reviews problems that can occur in the arterial and venous network. As pointed out in the first section on hy-

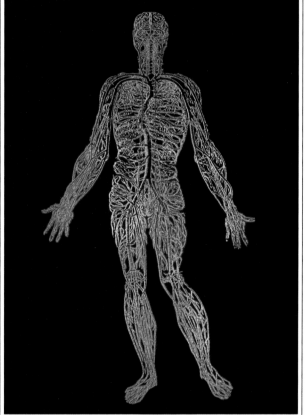

pertension, excessive pressure of blood flowing through the arteries rarely causes any symptoms. Yet, long-term high blood pressure can seriously damage several vital body organs, including the heart, kidneys, eyes, and brain. Detecting and controlling high blood pressure is one of the most important means of preventing heart disease and stroke. Hypertension is a condition that affects the entire arterial system

and the heart, but the arteries can also become diseased in a patchy, localized way. The second section of this chapter examines how atherosclerosis can narrow the major arteries in the trunk and legs, reducing blood flow to dangerously low levels. This narrowing may suddenly become more severe as a result of thrombosis (a blood clot forming inside an artery) or an embolism (blockage of a small artery by a moving blood clot). Other disorders discussed here include aneurysm (in which an artery balloons out and may burst) and inflammatory conditions such as temporal arteritis. New treatments are transforming the outlook for many arterial disorders. Drugs can reduce the risk of thrombosis and dissolve blood clots, and surgery can widen or reconstruct diseased vessels. One of the latest treatments is balloon angioplasty, a procedure in which a balloon catheter is inflated to flatten atheromatous plaques adhering to the inner lining of an artery. In many cases, this procedure proves successful in unblocking narrowed arteries, thus restoring the blood circulation. In the final section of this chapter, we examine disorders affecting the veins – the blood vessels that return blood to the heart. The development and treatment of varicose veins are also described.

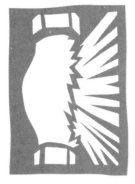

HYPERTENSION

HYPERTENSION IS THE TERM doctors use to describe blood pressure that is persistently abnormally high. About one in four Americans suffers from hypertension. It is important for hypertension to be detected and treated as early as possible because it can increase the risk of a heart attack, stroke, or other circulatory disease.

The blood is forced to circulate around the body by waves of pressure exerted by contractions of the heart. Using a sphygmomanometer, your doctor measures the pressure of your blood as it flows through the arteries. Two readings are recorded. The first, the systolic pressure, is taken as the heart contracts and the pressure is at its maximum. The second, the diastolic pressure, is taken at the point when the pressure reaches its minimum level. Blood pressure readings are usually recorded by rounding up or down to the nearest 5 millimeters of mercury (mm Hg). For example, a reading of 146 mm Hg (systolic) and 84 mm Hg (diastolic) would be recorded as a blood pressure of 145/85 mm Hg.

In any group of people, blood pressure readings vary among individuals in the same way that their height and weight measurements differ. Blood pressure is considered normal as long as it is within a particular range. The pres-

DO YOU HAVE HYPERTENSION?

In people who have hypertension, the blood pressure stays high during periods of rest. Hypertension is commonly defined as a resting blood pressure that gives a systolic reading on the sphygmomanometer of greater than 140 millimeters of mercury (mm Hg) and/or a diastolic reading greater than 90 mm Hg. The severity of high blood pressure is usually graded according to the diastolic value alone.

Severe hypertension
A consistent diastolic reading of greater than 120 mm Hg indicates severe hypertension; drug treatment is essential.

Mild hypertension
A consistent diastolic reading of between 95 and 105 mm Hg indicates mild hypertension, which should be promptly treated.

Moderately severe hypertension
This is defined as a consistent diastolic reading of between 105 and 120 mm Hg. Drug treatment is strongly recommended.

Borderline hypertension
This is a consistent diastolic reading of between 90 and 95 mm Hg. Preventive measures are recommended (see page 112).

Normal
A consistent diastolic reading of between 50 and 90 mm Hg is considered normal and healthy.

Hypotension
Hypotension (low blood pressure) is difficult to define since some young, healthy women have diastolic pressures as low as 50 mm Hg.

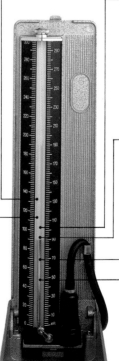

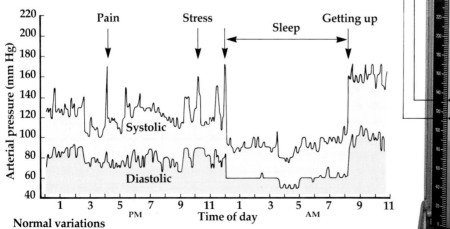

Normal variations
It is normal for your systolic and diastolic blood pressure readings to vary widely during the course of a day. Both readings are highest at the start of the day and during moments of stress or pain; they are lowest during sleep.

sure also goes up and down during the day, being at its highest during moments of stress, pain, or physical activity, and at its lowest during sleep.

It is normal for blood pressure to increase steadily with age as the artery walls become harder and less elastic. People over the age of 65 are much more likely to have high blood pressure readings than young, healthy adults.

RISK FACTORS

In the US, an estimated 58 million people have high blood pressure or take medication for high blood pressure. Only two thirds of those with high blood pressure know that it is high; only half of these people are taking medication. Hypertension is more common in the elderly, it is

WHO IS PRONE TO HYPERTENSION?

As the graph below shows, there is a parallel increase in the prevalence of hypertension in men and women between the ages of 30 and 40. After the age of 40, women become more prone to the development of hypertension. The reasons for this are unknown, but the hormonal changes associated with the menopause may be a contributing factor.

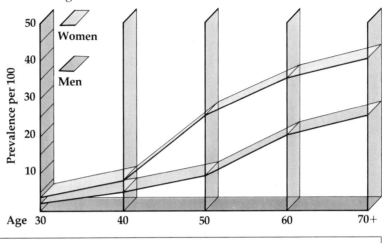

DOES YOUR HYPERTENSION HAVE A SPECIFIC CAUSE?

Only about 10 percent of cases of hypertension are caused by specific underlying diseases. Some of the most common causes of disease-related hypertension are shown below.

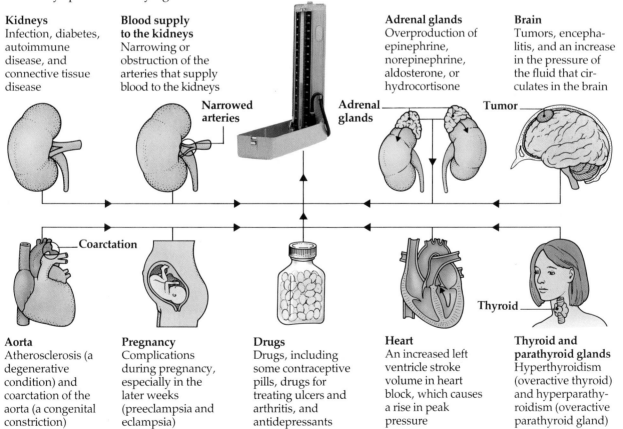

Kidneys
Infection, diabetes, autoimmune disease, and connective tissue disease

Blood supply to the kidneys
Narrowing or obstruction of the arteries that supply blood to the kidneys

Adrenal glands
Overproduction of epinephrine, norepinephrine, aldosterone, or hydrocortisone

Brain
Tumors, encephalitis, and an increase in the pressure of the fluid that circulates in the brain

Aorta
Atherosclerosis (a degenerative condition) and coarctation of the aorta (a congenital constriction)

Pregnancy
Complications during pregnancy, especially in the later weeks (preeclampsia and eclampsia)

Drugs
Drugs, including some contraceptive pills, drugs for treating ulcers and arthritis, and antidepressants

Heart
An increased left ventricle stroke volume in heart block, which causes a rise in peak pressure

Thyroid and parathyroid glands
Hyperthyroidism (overactive thyroid) and hyperparathyroidism (overactive parathyroid gland)

ASK YOUR DOCTOR
HYPERTENSION

Q **I am taking a drug for hypertension. Are there any foods or other drugs that I should avoid?**

A No food, or food additive, should interfere with your treatment. However, tell your doctor if you are taking any other prescription or over-the-counter drugs. Some of them can diminish or intensify the effect of your antihypertensive drug.

Q **My husband has been told he has hypertension. Does that mean he is under too much tension?**

A Hypertension is the medical term for persistently high blood pressure. Although people who are under a lot of stress and find it difficult to relax have a greater risk of high blood pressure, tension is not the only cause of the condition. Many people with hypertension have a relaxed lifestyle, and some people subjected to enormous stress do not have high blood pressure.

Q **I feel perfectly healthy, so why does my doctor want me to take drugs for high blood pressure?**

A Without treatment you run a much higher risk of having a serious complication, such as stroke or a heart attack, within the next few years.

Q **I am being treated for hypertension. I have heard that blood pressure goes up during exercise. Should I avoid it?**

A It is safe to continue aerobic exercises, such as brisk walking, as long as the exertion does not cause any symptoms. Avoid anaerobic exercises such as heavy lifting, which can cause your blood pressure to rise.

found more often in blacks than in whites, and it occurs more frequently in people with a history of hypertension in their family. Smoking, excessive alcohol consumption, being overweight, or being unable to relax increases the risk.

What causes hypertension?

In 90 percent of people with hypertension, no obvious cause can be found. In such cases, the condition is called essential hypertension. The remaining 10 percent of cases are caused by underlying diseases, as detailed on page 111.

How is hypertension investigated?

If your doctor finds that your blood pressure is persistently high, he or she will take your medical history, give you a thorough physical examination, and perform a series of tests. These may include blood and urine tests to check the function of the kidneys and to exclude diabetes. You may have a chest X-ray to detect any heart enlargement and an electrocardiogram to help detect signs of heart strain, enlargement, or coronary heart disease. You may also have an intravenous pyelogram (an X-ray of the urinary system) or an ultrasound scan to examine your kidneys for disease.

as detailed on page 111.

HOW CAN HYPERTENSION BE PREVENTED?

Hypertension, along with most disorders of the heart and circulation, is a condition that is less likely to occur if you follow these guidelines for an anticoronary life-style:
◆ Exercise regularly.
◆ Don't smoke.
◆ Drink alcohol in moderation.
◆ Keep your weight down.
◆ Choose a low-fat, high-fiber diet.
◆ Learn relaxation techniques.
◆ Have your blood pressure checked regularly – especially if you are taking contraceptive pills.

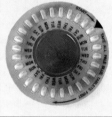

Weight control
As the graph (right) illustrates, if you lose weight, your diastolic blood pressure will be reduced by an average of 6 mm Hg for every 10 pounds of weight you lose. If you become overweight, your blood pressure rises accordingly. If you are overweight and need to lower your blood pressure, your doctor will begin by recommending ways to lose weight. Drug treatment is usually reserved for people whose blood pressure does not respond to weight loss.

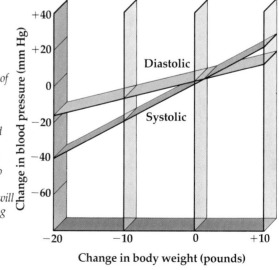

WHAT ARE THE EFFECTS OF HYPERTENSION?

Hypertension does not usually cause any symptoms; it can undermine your health without making you feel ill. You should have your blood pressure checked periodically – at least once every 5 years, and annually after age 55. Many employers offer on-site blood pressure testing. If yours does not, take advantage of the free testing offered at a health fair. Another means of scheduling a regular check is by donating blood; blood pressure is always tested before blood is taken.

If blood pressure is extremely high, it occasionally causes certain types of headache, nausea, tiredness, dizziness, or blurred vision. If you have any of these symptoms, your doctor will check your blood pressure, but the cause is much more likely to be another health problem.

Untreated hypertension increases your chances of a number of serious illnesses (see right). How likely they are to develop depends on the severity of the high blood pressure and the length of time that it has been abnormal.

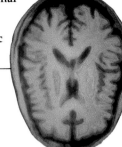

Cross-sectional brain scan obtained by magnetic resonance imaging

Brain
High pressure of the blood flowing through the arteries in the brain increases the risk of stroke. In severe cases, hypertension can cause mental confusion, seizures, and coma.

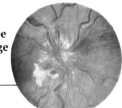

View of retina through ophthalmoscope showing damage caused by hypertension

Eyes
High blood pressure causes retinopathy (damage to the arteries in the retina). Examination of the retina with an ophthalmoscope can detect hypertension.

Angiogram showing coronary arteries that supply heart muscle

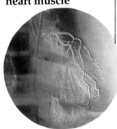

Heart
The heart strains and enlarges to overcome the resistance in the arteries, which is expressed as high blood pressure. This can lead to disorders such as angina, heart attack, stroke, and kidney and heart failure.

Angiogram showing blood supply to kidneys (outlined)

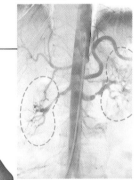

Kidneys
High blood pressure can cause thickening and hardening of the blood vessels in the kidneys and can lead to serious impairment of their function. Damage to the kidneys can aggravate certain types of hypertension.

Cross section of artery affected by atheroma

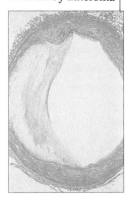

Blood vessels
Blood flowing through the aorta and other major arteries at a raised pressure for a prolonged period can reduce the elasticity of these vessels. At the same time, the process of atherosclerosis is accelerated.

TREATMENT FOR HYPERTENSION

Not everyone with hypertension needs drug treatment. If you are overweight, establishing normal weight may be all that is necessary to bring your blood pressure down. In some people, hypertension may respond to a reduction in the amount of salt in the diet. Drinking less alcohol and quitting smoking also help reduce blood pressure.

Medication for hypertension

If these measures have no effect, and your blood pressure stays above normal, your doctor may prescribe drug treatment (see ANTIHYPERTENSIVE DRUGS on page 127). People who have blood pressure that is extremely high or difficult to control may be treated with very potent drugs and their conditions may be monitored for a few days in a hospital.

How long does the treatment last?

Once you start drug treatment, you will probably need some form of medication to keep your blood pressure under control for the rest of your life. Checkups are important, and the time between each one depends on how stable your blood pressure has become. Never stop taking your antihypertensive medication without first checking with your doctor. Suddenly stopping your medication could cause a dramatic rise in your blood pressure and result in a serious complication, such as a seizure or stroke.

Are there any side effects?

Some people react poorly to a certain antihypertensive drug, but feel fine taking a different one. Occasionally the dose of the drug must be reduced because blood pressure has fallen too far. If you have any symptoms that you think may be occurring as a side effect of your antihypertensive medication, call your doctor for advice as soon as possible.

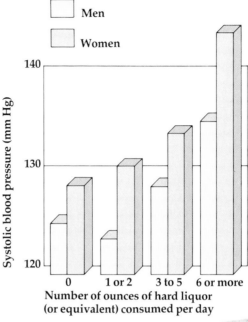

Number of ounces of hard liquor (or equivalent) consumed per day

☐ Men
▨ Women

Systolic blood pressure (mm Hg): 120, 130, 140

0   1 or 2   3 to 5   6 or more

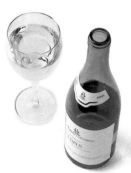

Alcohol consumption
As the graph (left) shows, the average systolic blood pressure increases sharply among men and women who regularly drink more than 2 ounces of hard liquor (or the equivalent) per day.

Smoking
The graphs (below) show how smoking causes a rise in blood pressure. The long-term effects of cigarette smoking on blood pressure have not been studied. But, apart from its repeated short-term effect, smoking

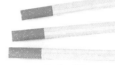

aggravates health problems, such as atherosclerosis, that may themselves cause hypertension.

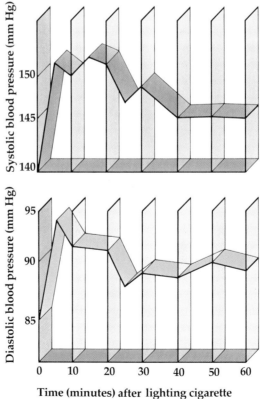

Systolic blood pressure (mm Hg): 140, 145, 150

Diastolic blood pressure (mm Hg): 85, 90, 95

0   10   20   30   40   50   60

Time (minutes) after lighting cigarette

SALT RESTRICTION

If you have hypertension, restricting your intake of salt and of salt-containing foods can reduce your diastolic blood pressure by an average of 5 mm Hg. Though not as beneficial as losing weight, restricting salt is an important part of any program designed to reduce hypertension without using drugs. In healthy people, there is insufficient evidence that reducing salt intake is useful as a preventive measure, unless salt intake is extremely high.

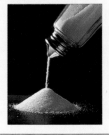

CASE HISTORY
HIGH BLOOD PRESSURE

GEORGE HAS NOT SEEN a doctor in more than 20 years. He regards himself as fit and healthy for a man in his 40s, although he smokes a pack of cigarettes a day and thinks he is a few pounds overweight. When one of his close friends about his age suddenly died of a heart attack, George made an appointment with a doctor for a checkup.

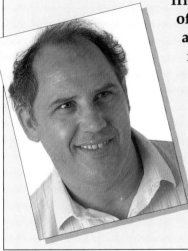

PERSONAL DETAILS
Name George Hopkins
Age 48
Occupation Blues musician
Family Father died of heart trouble in his 50s. Mother is well.

MEDICAL BACKGROUND
George last saw a doctor when he was 21, when he had an emergency appendectomy. Before that, he had only the usual childhood illnesses.

THE CONSULTATION
George tells his doctor that he has never suffered from chest pain or palpitations, but says he becomes breathless after running a few yards.

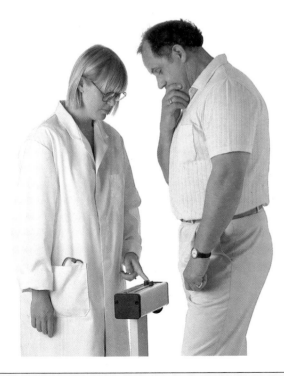

Weight problem
Like many people with hypertension, George was unaware that he gradually had become seriously overweight.

George's doctor finds that George has underestimated his weight problem. Although he is 6 feet tall, at 220 pounds George is at least 30 pounds over his ideal weight. His resting blood pressure is 165/100 mm Hg. Otherwise, the results of his examination are normal.

FURTHER INVESTIGATION
The doctor arranges for George to have a chest X-ray, an electrocardiogram, and a series of blood tests. All of the results are normal. A week later, the doctor checks George's blood pressure again and the result is as high as before.

THE DIAGNOSIS
George is suffering from MILD HYPERTENSION, which is probably caused by his excess weight.

THE TREATMENT
Since the blood pressure readings are only moderately raised, George does not require drug treatment. His doctor explains why George must work to lose some weight and, to help him stop smoking, the doctor prescribes nicotine gum.

THE OUTCOME
Forewarned by his friend's death, George quits smoking and is determined to lose weight. He walks 3 miles three times a week to rehearsals, a big improvement over his previous monthly games of golf. In addition, George drastically cuts the fat content of his meals, choosing leaner meats and plenty of fruits and vegetables. Within 2 months he loses 20 pounds and his blood pressure has come down to 145/85 mm Hg. His doctor congratulates him on markedly reducing his chances of suffering a heart attack and advises him to check his weight and blood pressure every 3 months.

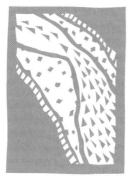

ARTERIAL DISORDERS

ATHEROSCLEROSIS AFFECTS NOT only the coronary arteries but also the entire arterial network, from the largest artery – the aorta – to the smallest arterioles. Arteries may also be affected by clot formation and inflammatory conditions. The term peripheral arterial disease is often used to refer to a range of disorders affecting the arteries other than those that supply the heart.

The arterial network is subject to a number of life-threatening disorders, several of which are caused by atherosclerosis and the formation of blood clots within the arterial channel. In addition, arteries may be affected by aneurysms (balloon-like swellings) and by a range of inflammatory diseases that can be just as serious as those caused by atherosclerosis.

THROMBOSIS

Thrombosis is the formation of a thrombus, or blood clot; it can take place inside an artery or a vein or in the heart itself. Blood clotting is an automatic, self-sealing process that occurs to prevent blood loss when a blood vessel is rup-

HOW DOES THROMBOSIS OCCUR?

The process of thrombosis (blood clot formation) is triggered when blood comes into contact with collagen fibers inside the arterial lining. Contact does not occur in healthy, intact arteries. A crack in an atheromatous plaque usually enables blood and collagen to come together. Once started, the clotting mechanism can create a blood clot that blocks the artery completely.

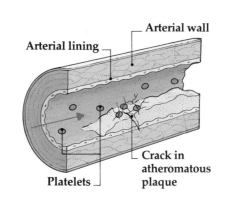

Arterial wall
Arterial lining
Crack in atheromatous plaque
Platelets

1 Blood entering a crack makes contact with collagen. The blood platelets begin to stick together and release chemicals. The chemicals help convert a soluble blood protein called fibrinogen into the insoluble protein fibrin.

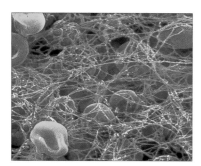

Fibrin
The fibrin strands bind platelets and red blood cells into a tight, integrated whole. The photograph clearly shows the structure of a blood clot.

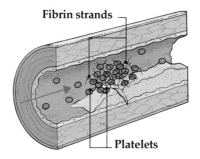

Fibrin strands
Platelets

2 Strands of fibrin become enmeshed in the clump of platelets to form a blood clot.

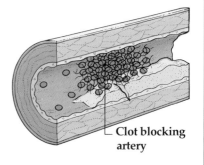

Clot blocking artery

3 The clotting causes more and more platelets to join the blood clot until it finally blocks the artery.

tured. However, if the clotting mechanism is triggered by damage to the inner lining of the blood vessel while the outer layer is still intact, the clot may obstruct the flow of blood through the vessel. Thrombosis in an artery is one of the main underlying causes of stroke (see page 121). Thrombosis in surface veins and deep veins is discussed on page 125.

How is thrombosis treated?

Thrombosis is treated with anticoagulant drugs (see page 136), which prevent clotting, and thrombolytic drugs (see page 137), which help dissolve clots that have already formed.

EMBOLISMS

Sometimes, part or all of a thrombus inside a blood vessel is detached and carried in the blood until it lodges elsewhere. The moving blood clot is called an embolus, and the blockage that it causes is called an embolism. Other materials can also be formed or released into the blood to cause a blockage, including debris from atheromatous plaques, cholesterol crystals, fat from the

WHERE DO EMBOLISMS OCCUR?

Embolisms can occur anywhere in the circulatory system. However, they are most commonly found at arterial bifurcations, where the sudden narrowing of the diameter of the artery along which an embolus is traveling can cause the embolus to block one or both of the arterial branches.

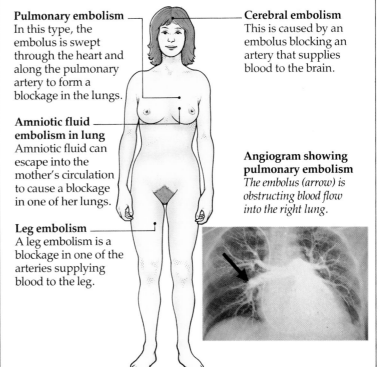

Pulmonary embolism
In this type, the embolus is swept through the heart and along the pulmonary artery to form a blockage in the lungs.

Cerebral embolism
This is caused by an embolus blocking an artery that supplies blood to the brain.

Amniotic fluid embolism in lung
Amniotic fluid can escape into the mother's circulation to cause a blockage in one of her lungs.

Leg embolism
A leg embolism is a blockage in one of the arteries supplying blood to the leg.

Angiogram showing pulmonary embolism
The embolus (arrow) is obstructing blood flow into the right lung.

HOW IS AN EMBOLISM TREATED?

Thrombolytic and anticoagulant drugs may be prescribed to treat an embolism. Otherwise, an operation called an embolectomy (below) may be required to remove the blockage.

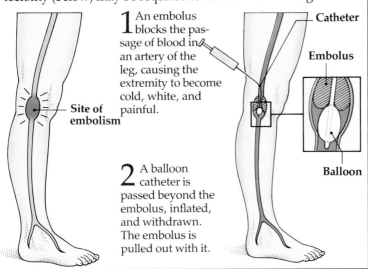

1 An embolus blocks the passage of blood in an artery of the leg, causing the extremity to become cold, white, and painful.

Site of embolism

2 A balloon catheter is passed beyond the embolus, inflated, and withdrawn. The embolus is pulled out with it.

Catheter

Embolus

Balloon

marrow of fractured bones, amniotic fluid from the uterus in pregnancy, and even large bubbles of air.

Do embolisms threaten life?

Some embolisms have serious effects. A large thrombus that has formed in a deep vein of the leg (see DEEP-VEIN THROMBOSIS on page 125) may break off and travel via the heart to the lungs, causing a blockage (pulmonary embolism) that may be fatal. Embolisms affecting the arteries that supply the brain usually originate in the large arteries near the heart. Thrombi from the left side of the heart, and matter from damaged and infected heart valves, may also cause cerebral embolism or stroke. In other cases, emboli may pass down the aorta to block the blood vessels to the intestines, kidneys, or legs.

SURGICAL PROCEDURES
BALLOON ANGIOPLASTY

BALLOON ANGIOPLASTY **can successfully treat arteries narrowed by atherosclerosis. The narrowed artery is widened by inserting a balloon at the tip of a catheter and then inflating it at the site of the blockage. The procedure was originally thought to work by squashing the atheromatous plaque into the wall of the artery, but it is now known that the plaque often actually cracks, allowing more room in the channel of the vessel.**

2 The guide wire is guided up the artery until it reaches the obstruction; its tip is then eased gently between the atheromatous plaques. The balloon catheter is then threaded over the guide wire, until the balloon at its tip is positioned at the site of obstruction.

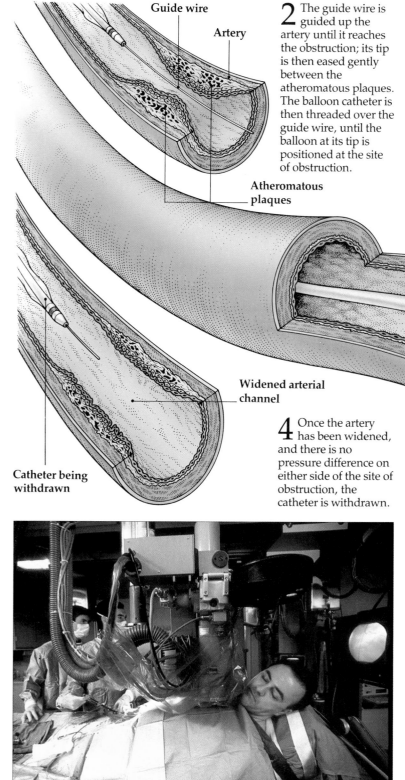

Guide wire

Artery

Atheromatous plaques

Widened arterial channel

Catheter being withdrawn

4 Once the artery has been widened, and there is no pressure difference on either side of the site of obstruction, the catheter is withdrawn.

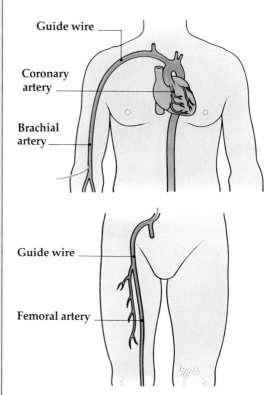

Guide wire

Coronary artery

Brachial artery

Guide wire

Femoral artery

1 Balloon angioplasty is performed in the operating suite of a hospital (right). If a coronary artery is to be cleared (top), an incision is made in the elbow to gain access to the brachial artery, through which a guide wire is pushed into the aorta and into the affected coronary artery. If an artery in the leg is to be unblocked (above), an incision is made in the groin to gain access to the femoral artery. Continuous imaging by X-rays or ultrasound is required to keep the guide wire on the right course.

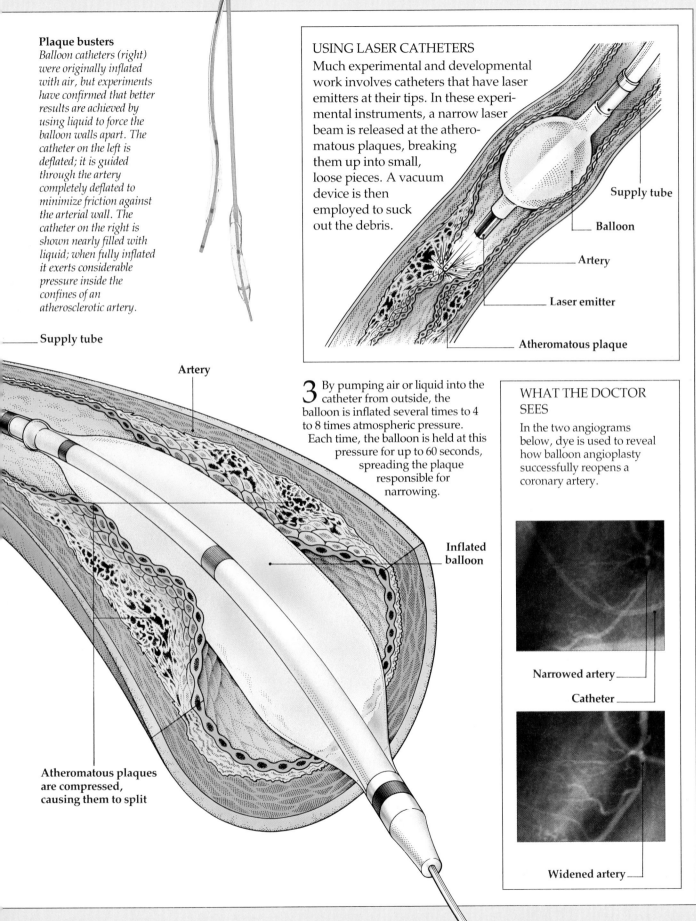

Plaque busters
Balloon catheters (right) were originally inflated with air, but experiments have confirmed that better results are achieved by using liquid to force the balloon walls apart. The catheter on the left is deflated; it is guided through the artery completely deflated to minimize friction against the arterial wall. The catheter on the right is shown nearly filled with liquid; when fully inflated it exerts considerable pressure inside the confines of an atherosclerotic artery.

Supply tube

Artery

Supply tube

USING LASER CATHETERS

Much experimental and developmental work involves catheters that have laser emitters at their tips. In these experimental instruments, a narrow laser beam is released at the atheromatous plaques, breaking them up into small, loose pieces. A vacuum device is then employed to suck out the debris.

Supply tube

Balloon

Artery

Laser emitter

Atheromatous plaque

3 By pumping air or liquid into the catheter from outside, the balloon is inflated several times to 4 to 8 times atmospheric pressure. Each time, the balloon is held at this pressure for up to 60 seconds, spreading the plaque responsible for narrowing.

Inflated balloon

Atheromatous plaques are compressed, causing them to split

WHAT THE DOCTOR SEES

In the two angiograms below, dye is used to reveal how balloon angioplasty successfully reopens a coronary artery.

Narrowed artery

Catheter

Widened artery

MONITOR YOUR SYMPTOMS
FEELING FAINT AND FAINTING

Fainting is a loss of consciousness due to an insufficient supply of oxygen reaching the brain. Before fainting, people usually feel weak or unsteady, and the skin may become cold and clammy. In most cases, fainting attacks are no cause for concern. If you faint frequently or have other symptoms, consult your doctor.

WARNING

There is usually no reason to worry if a person loses consciousness briefly. However, if unconsciousness lasts longer or breathing slows or becomes noisy or irregular, get medical help immediately.

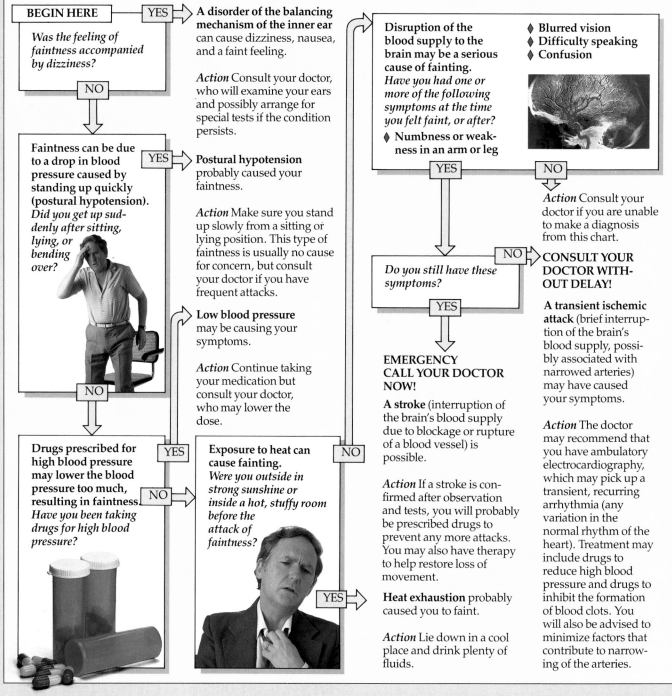

BEGIN HERE — YES →

Was the feeling of faintness accompanied by dizziness?

NO

A disorder of the balancing mechanism of the inner ear can cause dizziness, nausea, and a faint feeling.

Action Consult your doctor, who will examine your ears and possibly arrange for special tests if the condition persists.

Faintness can be due to a drop in blood pressure caused by standing up quickly (postural hypotension). *Did you get up suddenly after sitting, lying, or bending over?* — YES →

NO

Postural hypotension probably caused your faintness.

Action Make sure you stand up slowly from a sitting or lying position. This type of faintness is usually no cause for concern, but consult your doctor if you have frequent attacks.

Low blood pressure may be causing your symptoms.

Action Continue taking your medication but consult your doctor, who may lower the dose.

Drugs prescribed for high blood pressure may lower the blood pressure too much, resulting in faintness. *Have you been taking drugs for high blood pressure?* — YES

NO →

Exposure to heat can cause fainting. *Were you outside in strong sunshine or inside a hot, stuffy room before the attack of faintness?* — NO

YES →

Disruption of the blood supply to the brain may be a serious cause of fainting. *Have you had one or more of the following symptoms at the time you felt faint, or after?*

♦ **Numbness or weakness in an arm or leg**
♦ **Blurred vision**
♦ **Difficulty speaking**
♦ **Confusion**

YES — NO

Action Consult your doctor if you are unable to make a diagnosis from this chart.

Do you still have these symptoms? — NO →

CONSULT YOUR DOCTOR WITHOUT DELAY!

YES

EMERGENCY CALL YOUR DOCTOR NOW!

A stroke (interruption of the brain's blood supply due to blockage or rupture of a blood vessel) is possible.

Action If a stroke is confirmed after observation and tests, you will probably be prescribed drugs to prevent any more attacks. You may also have therapy to help restore loss of movement.

Heat exhaustion probably caused you to faint.

Action Lie down in a cool place and drink plenty of fluids.

A transient ischemic attack (brief interruption of the brain's blood supply, possibly associated with narrowed arteries) may have caused your symptoms.

Action The doctor may recommend that you have ambulatory electrocardiography, which may pick up a transient, recurring arrhythmia (any variation in the normal rhythm of the heart). Treatment may include drugs to reduce high blood pressure and drugs to inhibit the formation of blood clots. You will also be advised to minimize factors that contribute to narrowing of the arteries.

STROKE

Stroke is a general term that covers any of the consequences of a loss of brain function. Disease affecting the arteries in the brain (cerebrovascular disease) may cause stroke in several ways.

Transient ischemic attacks

Cerebrovascular disease may cause a transient ischemic attack, a brief, but often recurrent, loss of brain function that appears suddenly and lasts from a minute to a few hours. It is thought to be due to a transient spasm or temporary blockage of small arteries in the brain by clumps of platelets. The attacks tend to affect elderly people and usually involve only one side of the brain. They may cause loss of feeling on one side of the body; loss of vision in one eye or loss of half of the field of vision in both eyes; difficulty reading, choosing a word, or understanding speech; vertigo; and confusion.

Major stroke

A more severe manifestation of cerebrovascular disease is stroke. A stroke is similar to a transient ischemic attack, but its effects are more severe because it is usually caused by a blood clot or embolism that completely blocks an artery in the brain. In a stroke, part of the brain tissue dies, but the tissue surrounding it often survives. A stroke also may be caused by rupture of a blood vessel in the brain (a cerebral hemorrhage). The damaged artery may be inside the brain, between the brain and its surrounding membranes (the meninges), or beneath the brain substance itself.

How is stroke treated?

If a transient ischemic attack or a stroke is caused by clumping of platelets or by a thrombus or embolism, aspirin and anticoagulant drugs are used to help prevent a recurrence. Some cerebral hemorrhages, and some cerebral thrombi and emboli, may be treated by surgery.

BUERGER'S DISEASE

Buerger's disease affects the small and medium arteries, veins, and nerves, commonly in the legs. It is characterized by inflammation, formation of a thrombus, and vascular obstruction. The parts beyond the obstruction become cold, numb, and painful, and there is intermittent claudication (see page 122). A lack of blood supply leads, in many cases, to skin ulcers and progressive gangrene, which starts at the toes and fingers. The condition may be suspected when the previously mentioned symptoms and signs occur in men between 20 and 40 years of age who smoke cigarettes. Victims of the disease who stop smoking completely and permanently sometimes make a partial recovery.

WHAT ARE THE CAUSES OF STROKE?

There are three causes of stroke. In cerebral thrombosis and cerebral embolism, death of brain tissue is caused by blockage of an artery. In hemorrhage, the damage is caused by bleeding into or over the surface of the brain.

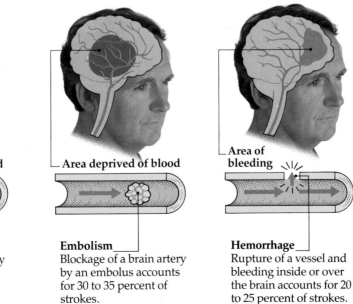

Area deprived of blood

Area deprived of blood

Area of bleeding

Thrombosis
Blockage of a brain artery by a thrombus accounts for 40 to 50 percent of strokes.

Embolism
Blockage of a brain artery by an embolus accounts for 30 to 35 percent of strokes.

Hemorrhage
Rupture of a vessel and bleeding inside or over the brain accounts for 20 to 25 percent of strokes.

WHAT CAUSES AN ANEURYSM?

A common aneurysm is a ballooning caused by blood pressing against a weakness in the arterial wall. A dissecting aneurysm occurs when blood escapes into the wall of the artery, causing it to bulge, thin, and sometimes rupture.

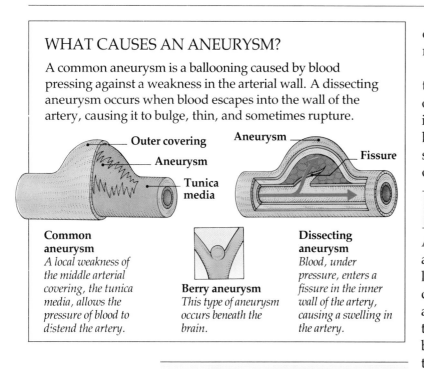

Outer covering
Aneurysm
Tunica media
Aneurysm
Fissure

Common aneurysm
A local weakness of the middle arterial covering, the tunica media, allows the pressure of blood to distend the artery.

Berry aneurysm
This type of aneurysm occurs beneath the brain.

Dissecting aneurysm
Blood, under pressure, enters a fissure in the inner wall of the artery, causing a swelling in the artery.

deprived muscle, which stimulates nerve endings and causes pain.

The treatment is to stop smoking and to exercise regularly. Although pain may occur during exercise, it stops after resting; exercising can then be resumed. Balloon angioplasty (see page 118) or bypass surgery has been successfully used to open up certain vessels.

ANEURYSMS

An aneurysm is a ballooning out of an artery. This protrusion may result from a lifelong weakness in the artery, or from a disease or injury that has weakened the arterial walls. It is usually necessary to treat aneurysms by surgery, preferably before the arterial wall thins to the point that rupture is imminent.

Where are aneurysms found?

Small aneurysms, known as berry aneurysms, commonly occur on the circle of Willis, a circle of arteries on the underside of the brain. Berry aneurysms are often congenital (present from birth). They occur where the arteries divide, either on the circle of Willis itself or on its branches, and they often burst in comparatively young adults. Warning signs are a drooping eyelid, a dilated pupil, or double vision from paralysis of movement of one eye. Rupture of the aneurysm causes serious bleeding, called a subarachnoid hemorrhage, which is a significant cause of stroke in people between the ages of 25 and 50.

INTERMITTENT CLAUDICATION

Intermittent claudication is similar to angina in that it is a pain – not a disease – that usually occurs only after exercise. The pain of intermittent claudication, which may be felt in the buttock, thigh, calf muscles, or arch of the foot, occurs after walking a certain distance.

Intermittent claudication is caused by a restriction in the blood supply to the legs, usually as a result of atherosclerosis. Exercise creates a demand for glucose and oxygen that cannot be met because the blockage prevents sufficient blood from reaching the muscle tissue. As a result, lactic acid is produced by the

Raynaud's phenomenon
Spasm of the arteries in the hands or feet, causing successive white, blue, and red coloration, is an occupational disorder of people who use vibrating tools such as pneumatic drills and chain saws. People whose hands are subjected to repeated trauma, such as pianists and typists, also suffer from the phenomenon.

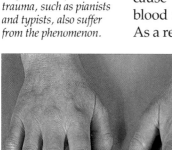

Ulcers
An insufficient arterial blood supply to, or an inadequate venous drainage from, an area of tissue can result in ulcers, such as the leg ulcers shown at right. The ulcers occur because the tissue is not receiving the oxygen and nutrients it requires for healing to take place after minor damage.

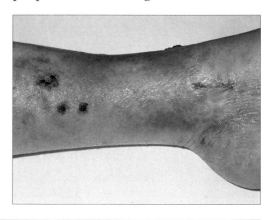

WHAT IS TEMPORAL ARTERITIS?

Temporal arteritis is an inflammatory condition that usually affects the temporal artery (below).

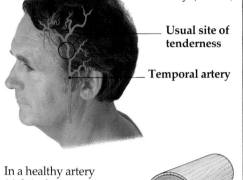

Usual site of tenderness

Temporal artery

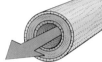

In a healthy artery (right), there is nothing to interrupt the smooth flow of blood.

Temporal arteritis thickens the arterial wall, severely restricting the blood flow (left).

The second major site for aneurysms is the aorta, the body's largest artery. The protrusion may take the form of a dissecting aneurysm, which progressively splits the wall of the aorta. Most people are unaware that they have an aortic aneurysm until either a pulsating mass is felt in the abdomen or a sudden, fatal rupture occurs. Aortic aneurysms must be treated by surgery to remove the affected part of the aorta and replace it with a length of artificial tubing.

TEMPORAL ARTERITIS

This dangerous condition causes segments of the arteries to become inflamed, thickening the arterial wall and narrowing the channel inside. Temporal arteritis can affect almost any artery in the body but it is especially common in the arteries that serve the head. The ophthalmic artery, which supplies the eye with blood, may be blocked, resulting in permanent blindness.

Temporal arteritis seldom affects people under 50 and the incidence rises with age. The cause is unknown. The condition causes severe headache, extreme tenderness over the arteries of the temple, a low fever, loss of appetite, and weakness. Temporal arteritis requires immediate treatment with large doses of corticosteroid drugs.

RAYNAUD'S DISEASE

Raynaud's disease is an arterial disorder marked by spasm of the small arteries of the fingers and toes in response to cold or emotional upset. It is called Raynaud's phenomenon if the spasm can be attributed to an underlying cause, such as rheumatoid arthritis. It is called Raynaud's disease if the cause is unknown.

The spasm closes off the blood supply, causing the skin to turn white from loss of blood. The blood remaining in the area soon loses its hemoglobin and becomes blue; when the spasm passes and the part is warmed, fresh blood returns to the area and turns it red. The spasm can last from a few minutes to a few hours.

How is it treated?

Treatment is directed at the underlying cause if it is known. Otherwise the affected parts should be kept warm and drugs such as sympatholytics (see page 133) and calcium channel blockers (see page 132) may be prescribed to reduce the tendency to spasm. Nicotine makes the spasm worse.

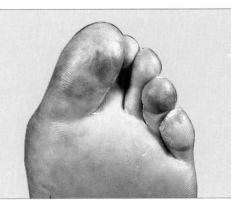

GANGRENE

Gangrene is death of tissue. The affected area can range from the tip of a finger to a complete limb. The first sign of gangrene is a blackening of the affected part.

Gangrene usually occurs after a period of slow, progressive reduction in blood supply to the part. At first there may be pain only during exertion – called intermittent claudication. As the condition worsens, there may be severe and persistent pain at rest. The affected part becomes cold and numb, and the skin is often dry and scaly. Eventually, ulceration occurs, usually on the toes or heels. Gangrene may be thwarted if improvement in the circulation is achieved during the early stages, thus preventing the spread of the gangrene. Antibiotics are used to prevent bacterial infection. Otherwise, amputation of the part is vital.

Gangrene affecting the toes
There are two types of gangrene. Dry gangrene results from restriction of blood supply to the affected part. Wet gangrene develops when dry gangrene becomes infected or a wound is infected by certain bacteria.

VEIN DISORDERS

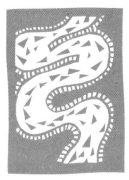

T HE WALLS OF VEINS are relatively weak compared to those of arteries. The most common disorder affecting them is varicose veins – swelling, lengthening, and twisting of veins. Veins may also be affected by clotting of the blood inside them, a condition known as thrombosis. Thrombosis in veins that lie close to the surface of the body rarely causes any problems, but clotting in a deep vein may have serious consequences.

Both varicose veins and vein thrombosis are, principally, disorders affecting the legs. The veins in the legs include the deep veins, which are embedded in muscle and carry most of the returning blood upward to the heart, and the superficial veins, which lie near the surface. Blood flows from the surface veins to the deep veins via perforating veins.

VARICOSE VEINS

The column of blood in your veins extends from your feet to your heart. If it were not broken up into short segments by a series of valves, the blood would exert great pressure on the walls of the

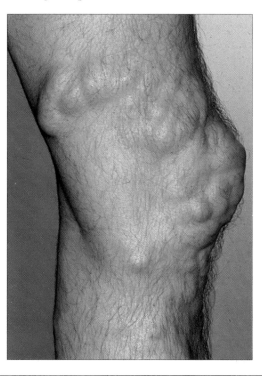

Appearance of varicose veins
This photograph of the knee area shows the typical knobby, twisted appearance of varicose veins. Varicose veins are very common, affecting about 15 percent of adults in the US.

lower veins. The valves allow blood to move only in an upward direction. If the valves fail, blood drains downward and pools in the superficial veins, causing swelling, twisting, and distortion. This condition is called varicose veins.

Who is at risk?
The reasons varicose veins develop are not known, but there is probably an inherited tendency to defective or absent valves. Contributing factors include being overweight or pregnant or standing for long periods. Varicose veins affect women far more commonly than men.

What are the symptoms and signs?
Varicose veins do not always cause pain. Cosmetic appearance may be the only problem, with affected veins appearing prominent, blue, and twisted. Other people experience severe aching and swelling in their legs due to stagnation of blood, which prevents efficient removal of waste products from the tissues. This symptom is usually exacerbated by standing for long periods and can be relieved only by raising the legs.

If very little blood is getting through to the tissues and they are starved of oxygen, skin ulcers may develop.

Treatment of varicose veins
In many cases, treatment of varicose veins involves wearing support stockings, walking regularly, and avoiding standing for too long. More severe cases

can be treated by injecting an irritant solution into the affected vein. This causes thrombosis and subsequent blockage of the vein, allowing other, healthy veins to take over the task of transporting blood. Alternatively, veins are treated surgically by tying off the perforating veins linking them to the deep veins and/or by stripping (see box).

VEIN THROMBOSIS

Thrombosis in a vein near the surface of the body is very common. The affected vein can be felt as a hard cord running under the skin. It may also be tender and slightly red but is no cause for concern.

Formation of a clot in the deeper, larger veins in the legs or pelvis (deep-vein thrombosis) may be more serious. Such a clot may be carried in the veins to the pulmonary artery, which leads from the heart to the lungs. At the point where the pulmonary artery narrows into smaller branches, the clot will cause obstruction (pulmonary embolism). If the clot is large enough, or extends far enough, to cut off most of the blood supply to the lungs, the outcome may be fatal.

SURGICAL PROCEDURES
STRIPPING A VARICOSE VEIN

SURGICAL STRIPPING **of varicose veins is reserved for cases in which the valves of the main superficial veins are known to be malfunctioning or in which there are skin ulcers.**

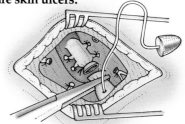

Site of incision

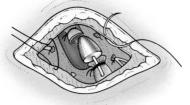

1 Through an incision in the groin, the greater saphenous vein is exposed and, with its four branches, cut and tied off.

2 A wire is inserted into a hole made in the top of the vein. It is fed through the vein to the calf or ankle and brought out through a small incision.

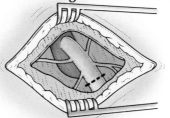

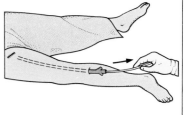

3 The upper end of the wire (which is specially shaped) is tied securely to the vein, and the groin incision is closed.

4 The vein is removed by pulling on the end of the wire protruding through the lower incision.

DEEP-VEIN THROMBOSIS

Clots, or thrombi, that form in a deep vein can provide a focus for more clotting. Eventually, clots may extend along the length of a vessel. The severity of symptoms and signs depends on their extent and location.

Posterior tibial vein
Anterior tibial vein

Femoral vein

Clots
Vein wall

Calf vein thrombosis
Clots in the calf and the veins behind the knee cause some pain, but usually little swelling.

Femoral vein thrombosis
Clots in the femoral and calf veins cause pain and swelling up to the area above the knee.

Iliofemoral vein thrombosis
If there are clots above the femoral vein, the whole leg may become painful and swollen.

PREVENTION OF DEEP-VEIN THROMBOSIS

Many deaths in hospitals are associated with deep-vein thrombosis leading to pulmonary embolism. To help reduce the risks, patients are urged to get out of bed as soon as possible after surgery and after such conditions as stroke. For those who cannot get up, a daily regimen of leg movements is started. Anticoagulant drugs are also routinely given.

DRUGS FOR THE HEART AND CIRCULATION

Many different drugs are available for treating heart and circulatory disorders. New drugs, and modifications of drugs already in use, are continuously being developed. This section is designed to help you understand why your doctor has prescribed a certain drug, how the drugs work, and what precautions you should take when using them.

Drug therapy is an important part of the treatment of many heart and circulatory disorders, especially angina (see page 74), heart rate and rhythm disorders (arrhythmias, see page 98), heart failure (see page 104), and many cases of hypertension (see page 110) where measures such as weight reduction have failed to control high blood pressure.

Modern heart drugs have powerful effects; certain procedures and precautions should always be followed (see box below).

Drug groups

The majority of drugs available to treat the heart and circulation fall into a small number of well-defined groups, according to their mode of action. On pages 128 to 137, each of these groups is reviewed (see box above). The text for each drug group describes how the drugs in that group work and why they are pre-

scribed, the typical dosages and forms in which the drugs are taken, special precautions for their use, common side effects, and what to do if a dose is missed or an overdose is taken. The more commonly prescribed drugs are also listed.

In addition, the table on the next page briefly reviews drug therapy for particular heart or circulatory disorders. For certain disorders, drug therapy may be recommended from any of several drug groups, or a combination of drugs may be prescribed. For example, heart failure is frequently treated with both a cardiac glycoside (e.g., digoxin) and a diuretic (e.g., furosemide). Some commonly prescribed drugs for certain disorders that do not belong to any of the drug groups on pages 128 to 137 are listed in the third column of the table.

Drug index

If you have been prescribed a drug for your heart or circulation and are not certain what it is for, the DRUG INDEX on pages 138 and 139 will help you identify to what drug group the drug belongs or what type of disorder it is used to treat.

PRECAUTIONS WITH PRESCRIBED DRUGS

◆ Be sure you understand your doctor's instructions regarding the dosage of each drug.

◆ Take the drugs as instructed. Do not take any more or less than the recommended dose.

◆ Talk to your doctor about any side effects of the drug treatment. If other side effects, or any severe side effects, develop, contact your doctor immediately.

◆ Report to your doctor any changes in the way a drug is affecting you (e.g., any loss of effectiveness in antiangina medication).

◆ Always inform your doctor if there is a chance you might become pregnant while you are taking the medication.

◆ Store drugs in a cool, dry place and out of the reach of children.

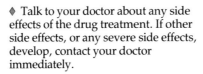
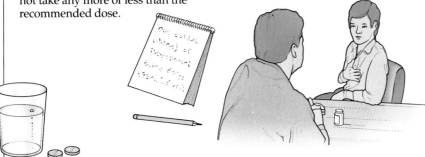
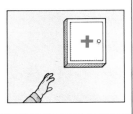

	PURPOSE	DRUGS COMMONLY USED	COMMENTS
ANTIANGINA DRUGS	To relieve pain by improving the blood supply to the heart muscle and/or by reducing the work load on the heart and thus its blood and oxygen requirements.	**Nitrates** (page 130) **Beta blockers** (page 129) **Calcium channel blockers** (page 132)	Nitrate tablets under the tongue are taken intermittently to relieve or prevent angina attacks. Beta blockers, calcium channel blockers, and long-acting nitrates are taken one or more times daily to prevent angina.

ANTIARRHYTHMIC DRUGS	To restore a normal heart rhythm by decreasing the excitability of the heart muscle, preventing unwanted electrical impulses from arising in the muscle, and stabilizing the conduction of normal impulses through the heart.	**Cardiac glycosides** (page 128)
		Beta blockers (page 129)
		Calcium channel blockers (page 132)
		Other drugs
		  Amiodarone
		  Disopyramide
		  Procainamide
		  Quinidine
		  Lidocaine
		  Tocainide
			Different antiarrhythmic drugs have varying effects and are used for different types of arrhythmias. Certain drugs may further disrupt heart rhythm under some circumstances and therefore are used only when the benefits outweigh the risks. Because the therapy is complex, it is usually supervised by a cardiologist.

DRUGS FOR HEART FAILURE	To restore and maintain the heart's pumping action and to reduce fluid collection in the lungs and tissues resulting from the heart failure.	**Cardiac glycosides** (page 128)
		Diuretics (page 134)
		ACE inhibitors (page 131)
		Sympatholytics (page 133)
		Other drugs
		  Amrinone
		  Dobutamine
		  Dopamine
			Cardiac glycosides strengthen the heart's contractions, diuretics reduce accumulation of fluid, and ACE inhibitors and sympatholytics reduce blood pressure and strain on the heart. Amrinone and dobutamine are generally reserved for patients who have severe heart failure or shock.

ANTIHYPERTENSIVE DRUGS	To lower blood pressure, either by widening the blood vessels (vasodilatation) or by reducing blood volume.	**Beta blockers** (page 129) **Diuretics** (page 134) **ACE inhibitors** (page 131) **Calcium channel blockers** (page 132) **Sympatholytics** (page 133) **Nitrates** (page 130) **Direct-acting vasodilators** Hydralazine, Minoxidil	Treatment may start with a single drug, often a diuretic, beta blocker, calcium channel blocker, or ACE inhibitor. If one drug does not reduce the pressure sufficiently, a combination may be used – sometimes a diuretic, a beta blocker, and a sympatholytic.

DRUGS FOR PERIPHERAL VASCULAR DISEASE	To improve blood flow through narrowed or blocked blood vessels by widening the vessels and making the blood less "sticky."	**Sympatholytics** (page 133)
		Calcium channel blockers (page 132)
		Other drugs
		  Pentoxifylline
		  Cyclandelate
		  Isoxsuprine
		Anticoagulants (page 136)
		Thrombolytics (page 137)
			Drugs that widen blood vessels (vasodilators), which include sympatholytics and calcium channel blockers, are sometimes used to treat peripheral arterial disorders. Anticoagulants and sometimes thrombolytics are used to treat deep vein thrombosis.

DRUGS FOR HYPERLIPIDEMIA	To lower the amount of lipids (fats) in the blood.	**Lipid-lowering drugs** (page 135)	These drugs help lower the risk of atherosclerosis and coronary heart disease in people with hyperlipidemia.
DRUGS USED AFTER A HEART ATTACK	To break up blood clots or reduce the risk of more blood clots in the coronary arteries.	**Thrombolytics** (page 137) **Antiplatelets** (page 136)	Other drugs, such as cardiac glycosides, beta blockers, or antiarrhythmics, may also be required after a heart attack.

127

CARDIAC GLYCOSIDES

Cardiac glycosides are also known as digitalis drugs. They are found in the leaves of plants of the foxglove family and have been refined or synthesized to be used in the treatment of certain heart disorders.

If you suffer from some types of heart rate or rhythm disorders (arrhythmia, page 98) or from heart failure (page 104), or if your heart muscle has been weakened by a heart attack (page 82), your doctor may prescribe cardiac glycosides. They are often prescribed in conjunction with diuretics (page 134) in the treatment of heart failure.

How do they work?

Cardiac glycosides slow down the passage of electrical impulses through the heart muscle, thus slowing down a fast, erratic heartbeat. They also enhance muscle contraction, so the heart beats more powerfully and efficiently.

Are there some people who shouldn't take cardiac glycosides?

Your doctor will be cautious about prescribing these drugs if you have impaired kidney or liver function, or if you are pregnant or breast-feeding. Your blood will be monitored regularly during treatment with cardiac glycosides. If your blood level of potassium is low you will be given a potassium supplement to reduce any risk of altered rhythm caused by the interaction of low potassium and the drug.

How will the drugs affect me?

If you are taking cardiac glycosides to relieve the symptoms of heart failure, you should notice a fairly rapid improvement of symptoms such as breathlessness, ankle swelling, and fatigue. You may find that you need to pass urine more frequently because the improved efficiency of your heartbeat moves more blood to your kidneys; the fluid that had accumulated in your tissues is removed as urine.

Occasionally, people taking cardiac glycosides experience increased tiredness, confusion, and digestive disturbances such as loss of appetite, stomach pain, and nausea or vomiting. This is usually because too high a dose of the drug is being taken. Report any problems to your doctor so that he or she can check the level of the drug in your blood and adjust it if necessary.

How do I take the drugs?

You will take your cardiac glycosides in tablet, capsule, or liquid form, depending on the type prescribed. In an emergency you may be given an injection of the drug to produce a rapid effect. The frequency of your treatment may be influenced by the amount of the drug in your blood but will probably be once daily.

What happens if I miss a dose?

Generally, missing a dose does not cause problems; your doctor will tell you exactly what to do.

Would an overdose be dangerous?

Some cardiac glycosides are more potent than others. However, an overdose should always be treated as an emergency.

How long will I have to take the drugs?

Occasionally, cardiac glycosides are prescribed as a short-term treatment. However, you will probably need to take them indefinitely because they do not cure the underlying problem. The effect of the drug may decline with long-term use.

COMMONLY PRESCRIBED
CARDIAC GLYCOSIDES
Digitoxin
Digoxin
Deslanoside

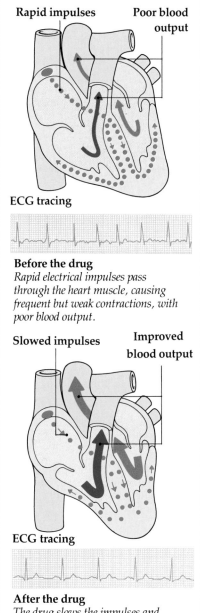

THE EFFECTS OF CARDIAC GLYCOSIDES

The heartbeat is triggered by electrical impulses that originate in the sinoatrial node – the heart's natural pacemaker. The electrical impulses then pass through the heart muscle, causing it to contract. Cardiac glycosides slow down the speed of these impulses and increase the force of each contraction.

Rapid impulses   Poor blood output

ECG tracing

Before the drug
Rapid electrical impulses pass through the heart muscle, causing frequent but weak contractions, with poor blood output.

Slowed impulses   Improved blood output

ECG tracing

After the drug
The drug slows the impulses and increases the force of the contractions, leading to improved blood output.

BETA BLOCKERS

If you suffer from angina (page 74), hypertension (page 110), a heart rhythm disorder (arrhythmia, page 98), or hypertrophic cardiomyopathy (page 93), your doctor may prescribe beta blockers. Beta blockers decrease your heart's oxygen requirements, reducing blood pressure and controlling certain kinds of rapid heartbeats. If you have had a heart attack, your doctor may give you a course of beta blockers to help prevent more damage to your heart muscle.

Are there some people who shouldn't take beta blockers?

Your doctor will prescribe beta blockers with caution if you have respiratory problems such as asthma or bronchitis, if you have poor circulation, or if you are pregnant. If you are diabetic, beta blockers may mask your normal warning symptoms of low blood sugar.

How will the drugs affect me?

If you suffer from angina or arrhythmia, you should notice an improvement in your condition within days or even hours after beginning treatment with beta blockers. If you are taking beta blockers for hypertension, you may not be aware of the drugs' beneficial effects.

Because the drugs may reduce circulation to the extremities, you may suffer from cold hands and feet. Occasionally, for the same reason, people taking beta blockers may experience lethargy, faintness, or temporary impotence.

How do I take the drugs?

You will take your beta blockers in either tablet or capsule form, between one and four times daily. Under some circumstances, beta blockers are administered in the hospital directly by injection.

What happens if I miss a dose?

Generally, missing a dose does not cause any problems; your doctor will tell you exactly what to do.

Would an overdose be dangerous?

An overdose of beta blockers requires immediate attention by your doctor and should always be treated as an emergency.

How long will I have to take the drugs?

Your doctor may suggest that you take the drugs indefinitely so that the beneficial effect is maintained.

You should not stop taking your beta blockers suddenly; this can cause a severe recurrence of the original problem. Your doctor may ask you to stop the drugs gradually before any scheduled surgery.

COMMONLY PRESCRIBED BETA BLOCKERS	
Acebutolol*	Nadolol
Atenolol*	Penbutolol
Carteolol	Pindolol
Labetalol	Propranolol
Metoprolol*	Timolol
* Cardioselective	

TYPES OF BETA BLOCKERS

There are two types of beta blockers – cardioselective and noncardioselective. Cardioselective beta blockers act primarily on the beta receptors in the heart muscle and not the airways, so they are generally preferable in treating people who also have respiratory problems. Noncardioselective beta blockers act on the receptors in the heart, airways, and blood vessels.

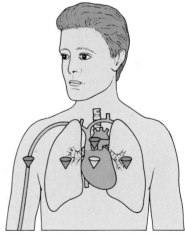

⏚ Parts of the body affected by cardioselective beta blockers.

▽ Parts of the body affected by noncardioselective beta blockers.

THE ACTION OF BETA BLOCKERS

Beta blockers attach themselves to, and thus block, the beta receptors in the heart, blood vessels, and other parts of the body. This stops the action of neurotransmitters that have been released by the sympathetic nervous system and that act on the beta receptors.

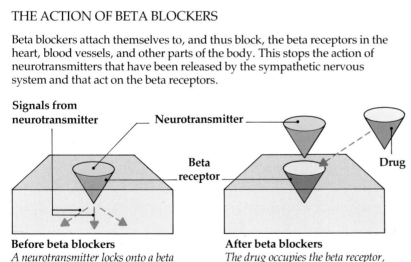

Before beta blockers
A neurotransmitter locks onto a beta receptor, carrying a signal that increases the heart rate or the strength of its contraction, or that constricts a blood vessel.

After beta blockers
The drug occupies the beta receptor, blocking the neurotransmitter and leading to a decrease in the heart rate or the strength of its contraction, or to dilation of blood vessels.

NITRATES

If you suffer from angina (page 74), your doctor may prescribe a nitrate drug. Nitroglycerin, the oldest of the nitrates, has been available since the end of the last century and is still considered a valuable drug for the treatment of angina.

How do they work?

Nitrate drugs relax the muscles surrounding the blood vessels so that they dilate (widen). This improves the flow of blood through the arteries around the heart and, by widening the blood vessels, promptly relieves an angina attack. If taken before an angina-provoking activity, nitroglycerin may prevent angina.

Are there some people who shouldn't take nitrates?

Your doctor will prescribe nitrates with caution if you have glaucoma, thyroid problems, or certain blood disorders, or if you are pregnant.

How will the drugs affect me?

Nitrate drugs can reduce both the pain and the frequency of your angina attacks, so you should notice an improvement soon after beginning treatment. Occasionally, people taking nitrate drugs experience side effects such as flushing, headache, dizziness, fainting, or edema; the dizziness and fainting are caused by a drop in blood pressure.

How do I take the drugs?

Nitrates are taken in different ways, depending on whether they are being used to treat or to prevent angina attacks. Methods of administration include tablets, capsules, injection, spray, ointment, and skin patches. They may be taken as needed, or several times daily as a preventive measure. Your doctor may suggest that you take your first dose while lying down, in case you feel dizzy. Don't stop taking drugs without consulting your doctor.

THE ACTION OF NITRATES

If the coronary arteries supplying the heart are narrowed, they restrict the heart's blood supply. As a result, when increased amounts of blood are needed, such as during exercise, the narrowed vessels fail to deliver the required increased volume. The characteristic pain of angina is produced by this lack of blood supply, which results in a lack of oxygen and the accumulation of waste products. Nitrates widen the coronary arteries and other blood vessels by inhibiting contraction of the muscle fibers in their walls. The blood supply to the heart is improved, and the work load on the heart reduced, relieving angina.

Before nitrate drugs
The coronary arteries are narrowed, restricting blood flow to the heart and causing pain as the heart works to maintain the circulation.

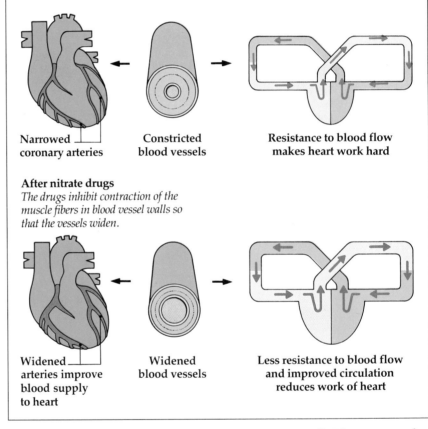

Narrowed coronary arteries   Constricted blood vessels   Resistance to blood flow makes heart work hard

After nitrate drugs
The drugs inhibit contraction of the muscle fibers in blood vessel walls so that the vessels widen.

Widened arteries improve blood supply to heart   Widened blood vessels   Less resistance to blood flow and improved circulation reduces work of heart

What happens if I miss a dose?

Generally, missing a dose does not cause any problems; your doctor will tell you exactly what to do.

Would an overdose be dangerous?

A single, unintentional extra dose is unlikely to cause problems, but a large overdose may cause dizziness, vomiting, severe headache, seizure, or loss of consciousness; it should be treated as a medical emergency.

How long will I have to take the drugs?

Nitrate drugs don't cure, so they may have to be taken indefinitely.

COMMONLY PRESCRIBED
NITRATES
Amyl nitrite
Erythrityl tetranitrate
Isosorbide dinitrate
Nitroglycerin
Pentaerythritol tetranitrate

ACE INHIBITORS

ACE inhibitors are a relatively new class of drugs used to treat heart disease; the first ACE inhibitor was introduced in 1981. If you suffer from hypertension (page 110), especially if you have had adverse reactions to other antihypertensive drugs, your doctor may prescribe ACE inhibitors. They are occasionally used with diuretics (page 134) to treat severe heart failure (page 104).

How do they work?
ACE stands for angiotensin-converting enzyme. ACE inhibitors prevent the action of a particular enzyme that promotes the constriction of blood vessel walls. As a result, the blood vessels dilate (widen), easing the flow of blood and reducing blood pressure.

Are there some people who shouldn't take ACE inhibitors?
Your doctor will prescribe ACE inhibitors with caution if you have impaired kidney or liver function, or if you are pregnant or breast-feeding. The possible adverse effects of the drugs may be more noticeable if you are elderly.

How will the drugs affect me?
ACE inhibitors rapidly control blood pressure, but because hypertension usually doesn't cause any symptoms you may not experience any noticeable benefits. Because the action of the drugs is so rapid, you should ideally take your first dose when you are lying down, in case you feel dizzy or faint. Similarly, when taking these drugs, it is wise to rise slowly from a sitting or lying position to prevent feelings of dizziness or faintness.

A cough may develop in some people who take these drugs. Digestive disturbances, such as loss of taste or appetite, nausea, vomiting, or diarrhea, may also occur. Captopril may also cause a minor rash in susceptible people.

ACE inhibitors also commonly affect the function of the kidneys, causing excessive fluid loss and general weakness. They sometimes also depress the action of the body's immune system, increasing susceptibility to infection.

How do I take the drugs?
Your doctor will prescribe ACE inhibitors in tablet form; the dose varies between one and three times daily. Because food inhibits the absorption of ACE inhibitors from the intestines, you may be advised to take the drugs before meals.

What happens if I miss a dose?
Generally, missing a dose does not cause any problems; your doctor will tell you exactly what to do.

Would an overdose be dangerous?
An overdose of ACE inhibitors may cause dizziness and fainting; seek medical advice if you notice any unusual symptoms or if a large overdose has been taken.

How long will I have to take the drugs?
ACE inhibitors don't cure the underlying condition, so you may need to take the drug indefinitely. Don't stop taking the drug without consulting your doctor; the original problem may recur.

COMMONLY PRESCRIBED
ACE INHIBITORS
Captopril
Enalapril
Lisinopril

THE ACTION OF ACE INHIBITORS

Before the drug
An enzyme is converting angiotensin I to angiotensin II.

After the drug
The action of the enzyme is blocked by the drug, so that angiotensin II cannot be formed.

Angiotensin I | Angiotensin II
Angiotensin-converting enzyme

Angiotensin I | Widened blood vessel
Drug blocks action of enzyme

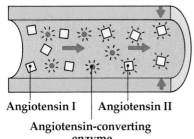

Angiotensin II | Constricted blood vessel

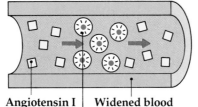

How ACE inhibitors work
Normally, an enzyme in the blood converts angiotensin I into angiotensin II, which constricts the muscles of the blood vessel walls (left, above and below). ACE inhibitors block the action of this enzyme so that angiotensin II is not formed, thus allowing the blood vessels to widen (above).

CALCIUM CHANNEL BLOCKERS

Calcium channel blockers are useful for treating many kinds of heart and circulation disorders. They help prevent attacks of angina (page 74) and regulate the heartbeat in heart rate and rhythm disorders (arrhythmias, page 98); they also improve the circulation, which is useful in treating some arterial disorders (page 116) and hypertension (page 110). Because they reduce the work load of the heart, they may be prescribed for heart failure (page 104).

How do they work?

Calcium channel blockers impede the flow of calcium into the muscles surrounding blood vessels so that the blood vessels are dilated (widened). As a result, the effort needed for the heart to pump blood around the body is also reduced.

Are there some people who shouldn't take calcium channel blockers?

Your doctor will prescribe these drugs with caution if you have unstable blood pressure, impaired kidney or liver function, or if you are pregnant or breast-feeding. Unlike beta blockers, calcium channel blockers can be given with less concern to people with asthma.

How will the drugs affect me?

If you suffer from angina, calcium channel blockers will reduce the frequency of your attacks, but only some types work rapidly enough to relieve the pain of an attack itself. Your circulation will improve, which is why these drugs sometimes help people who suffer from Raynaud's disease (page 123).

Calcium channel blockers may cause headache, nausea, edema, constipation, flushing, or lethargy. Occasionally, they cause dizziness; if you are affected in this way, do not drive or drink alcohol.

How do I take the drugs?

You will take your calcium channel blockers in tablet or capsule form. The drug will be taken between one and four times daily, depending on how long the dose remains active.

What happens if I miss a dose?

Generally, missing a dose does not cause any problems; your doctor will tell you what to do.

Would an overdose be dangerous?

A single extra dose is unlikely to cause problems, but several extra doses may cause dizziness and fainting. Seek medical advice if you notice any unusual symptoms or if a large overdose has been taken.

How long will I have to take the drugs?

While calcium channel blockers improve certain conditions dramatically (such as severe arrhythmias, angina, hypertension, and, in some instances, migraine), they generally cannot cure the underlying problem, so they may need to be taken indefinitely. In arterial disease, the beneficial effects may continue after use of the drug is stopped.

COMMONLY PRESCRIBED CALCIUM CHANNEL BLOCKERS	
Diltiazem	Nimodipine
Nicardipine	Verapamil
Nifedipine	

THE ACTION OF CALCIUM CHANNEL BLOCKERS

The movement of calcium into the muscle fibers in blood vessel walls causes the muscle fibers, which are arranged in a circular fashion, to contract and so narrow the blood vessels. Calcium channel blockers prevent the movement of calcium across the membranes that line the cells so that the muscles are unable to contract and the blood vessels widen. Calcium channel blockers also slow the passage of electrical impulses through heart muscle, which helps correct certain types of arrhythmias.

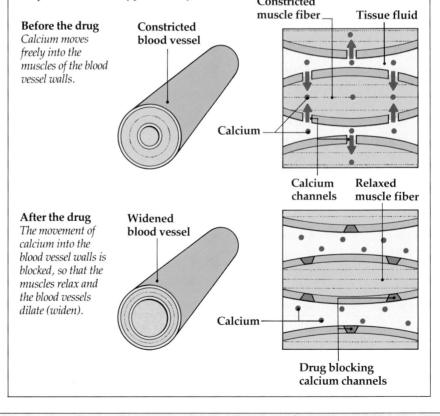

Before the drug
Calcium moves freely into the muscles of the blood vessel walls.

Constricted blood vessel

Constricted muscle fiber

Tissue fluid

Calcium

Calcium channels

Relaxed muscle fiber

After the drug
The movement of calcium into the blood vessel walls is blocked, so that the muscles relax and the blood vessels dilate (widen).

Widened blood vessel

Calcium

Drug blocking calcium channels

SYMPATHOLYTICS

If you suffer from moderate to severe hypertension (page 110), your doctor may prescribe a sympatholytic drug. These drugs are often prescribed with a diuretic (page 134), and sometimes a beta blocker (page 129) when the response to a single drug is considered inadequate. Sympatholytics may also be prescribed in cases of Raynaud's disease (page 123) and some cases of heart failure (page 104).

How do they work?
Sympatholytics are vasodilator drugs; they dilate (widen) the blood vessels in many parts of the body so that blood pressure is reduced. They achieve this effect by decreasing or blocking the activity of the sympathetic nervous system, which normally acts to constrict blood vessels in most parts of the body.

Some sympatholytics act on sympathetic nervous system control centers in the brain; others block the transmission of signals through sympathetic nerve pathways, or block the signals from having an effect on blood vessel walls.

Are there some people who shouldn't take sympatholytics?
Your doctor will prescribe sympatholytics with caution if you have impaired kidney or liver function, diabetes, a stomach ulcer or respiratory disorder, or if you are pregnant. You may not be prescribed sympatholytics to treat hypertension if you are suffering from some forms of heart disease.

Sympatholytics interact with many other kinds of drugs, so be sure to tell your doctor if you are taking any other prescribed or over-the-counter medication.

How will the drugs affect me?
Because hypertension tends not to cause any symptoms, you may not

THE ACTION OF SYMPATHOLYTICS

Normally, messages from the sympathetic nervous system travel to muscle fibers in the blood vessel walls and cause them to contract, which narrows the blood vessels. Sympatholytics reduce or block these nerve signals, so that the blood vessels widen.

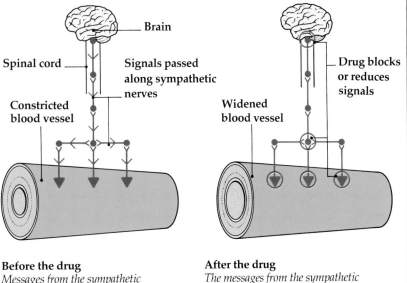

Before the drug
Messages from the sympathetic nervous system cause the muscles of the blood vessel walls to contract, narrowing the blood vessels.

After the drug
The messages from the sympathetic nervous system are reduced or blocked, allowing the blood vessels to widen.

notice that your blood pressure has been brought under control. If you have been having headaches as a result of hypertension, the situation will slowly improve.

Some people taking sympatholytics experience a dry mouth or stuffy nose, fatigue or drowsiness, or digestive disturbance such as nausea or diarrhea. These side effects usually diminish within 4 to 6 weeks. Dry mouth can be relieved by chewing gum or frequent rinsing of the mouth with water.

If your blood pressure drops too low, it may make you feel dizzy. Do not stand for prolonged periods in one position, and avoid alcohol and hot showers or baths. Also, avoid getting up too quickly from lying down or sitting positions.

How do I take the drugs?
Generally, sympatholytics are taken in tablet form. The frequency of your treatment will be between one and four times daily.

What happens if I miss a dose?
Generally, missing a dose does not cause any problems; your doctor will tell you exactly what to do.

Would an overdose be dangerous?
Some sympatholytics are more potent than others, but an overdose should be treated as an emergency.

How long will I have to take the drugs?
Sympatholytics cannot cure hypertension, so you will probably have to take the drugs indefinitely. Never stop taking them without first checking with your doctor.

COMMONLY PRESCRIBED SYMPATHOLYTICS	
Clonidine	Methyldopa
Guanabenz	Prazosin
Guanadrel	Reserpine
Guanethidine	Terazosin
Guanfacine	

THE ACTION OF DIURETICS

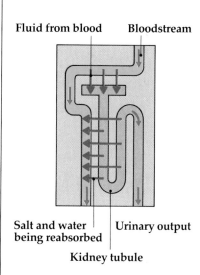

Fluid from blood　**Bloodstream**

Salt and water being reabsorbed　**Urinary output**

Kidney tubule

Before the drug
Inside the kidneys, fluid (water, waste products, and salt) is absorbed from the blood and passes down the kidney tubules. Much of the salt and water is reabsorbed into the blood. The rest of the water and waste products pass out as urine.

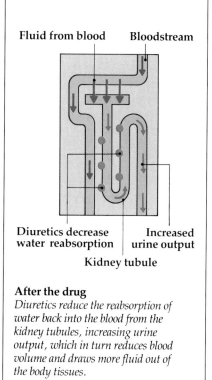

Fluid from blood　**Bloodstream**

Diuretics decrease water reabsorption　**Increased urine output**

Kidney tubule

After the drug
Diuretics reduce the reabsorption of water back into the blood from the kidney tubules, increasing urine output, which in turn reduces blood volume and draws more fluid out of the body tissues.

DIURETICS

If you have excess fluid in your body as a result of heart failure (page 104), or if you are suffering from hypertension (page 110), your doctor may prescribe a diuretic drug. All diuretics reduce the blood volume and therefore lower blood pressure and ease the heart's work load.

How do they work?

Diuretics interfere with the action of the kidneys to reduce the amount of water reabsorbed into the bloodstream. As a result, more fluid is drawn out of the tissues and expelled as urine. There are three common types of diuretic drugs – thiazide, loop, and potassium-sparing. Each works on a different part of the small tubes (tubules) in the kidneys.

Are there some people who shouldn't take diuretics?

Your doctor will prescribe diuretics with caution if you have gout or diabetes. Thiazide and loop diuretics can cause excessive loss of potassium from the body, which can have toxic effects. If your doctor believes there is a risk of potassium depletion, you may be prescribed a potassium-sparing diuretic as well as, or instead of, a thiazide or loop diuretic. Alternatively, a potassium supplement may be prescribed with a thiazide or loop diuretic.

How will the drugs affect me?

If you have edema or breathlessness, you should notice an improvement soon after you start taking your diuretic. You will need to urinate more frequently and, with loop diuretics, you may initially feel dizzy. Some diuretics cause leg cramps or temporary impotence, and some may cause nausea.

How do I take the drugs?

Diuretics are usually taken in tablet form, although a diuretic may be injected for a more rapid effect. The frequency of the drug will depend on the drug being taken.

What happens if I miss a dose?

Take the missed dose as soon as you remember. If you take one tablet daily and you remember you missed it near the end of the day, skip that dose and begin your scheduled dose again the following morning.

Would an overdose be dangerous?

An unintentional, extra dose of a diuretic is unlikely to cause major problems. If it is a large overdose, or if you notice any unusual symptoms, seek medical advice.

How long will I have to take the drugs?

Diuretics don't cure your underlying condition, so you may need to take them indefinitely. Never stop taking the diuretics without checking with your doctor.

COMMONLY PRESCRIBED DIURETICS

Thiazide and related diuretics
Bendroflumethiazide
Chlorothiazide
Chlorthalidone
Cyclothiazide
Flumethiazide
Hydrochlorothiazide
Hydroflumethiazide
Indapamide
Methyclothiazide
Metolazone
Polythiazide
Quinethazone
Trichlormethiazide

Loop diuretics
Bumetanide
Ethacrynic acid
Furosemide

Potassium-sparing diuretics
Amiloride
Spironolactone
Triamterene

LIPID-LOWERING DRUGS

People with hyperlipidemia (high levels of fats in the blood) are at high risk of atherosclerosis. If you suffer from hyperlipidemia, especially if you are diabetic or have circulatory disorders or a family history of heart attacks, treatment with a low-fat diet alone is unlikely to be effective. To bring down the level of fats in your blood, your doctor may prescribe lipid-lowering drugs.

How do they work?

There are two main types of lipid-lowering drugs – those that act on the liver and those that act on the bile salts (see box).

Are there some people who shouldn't take lipid-lowering drugs?

Your doctor will prescribe lipid-lowering drugs with caution if you have impaired kidney or liver function, if you have jaundice or gallstones, or if you have certain problems with your digestive tract.

How will the drugs affect me?

Because hyperlipidemia does not cause noticeable symptoms, you probably will not be aware of the beneficial effects of the drug. However, the lipid-lowering drug should prevent more buildup of atheroma in your arteries.

The drugs may cause digestive disturbance, which should improve as treatment continues. Certain drugs may also increase your susceptibility to gallstones.

How do I take the drugs?

Lipid-lowering drugs may come as tablets or capsules, or as powders to be mixed with juice or soft food. The frequency of treatment is between one and four times daily.

What happens if I miss a dose?

If you miss a dose of your drug, take it when you remember.

DRUGS THAT ACT ON THE LIVER

These drugs alter the enzyme activity in the liver to block the conversion of fatty acids to lipids. Ultimately, this action reduces the level of lipids in the blood, which can be lifesaving for people who have hyperlipidemia.

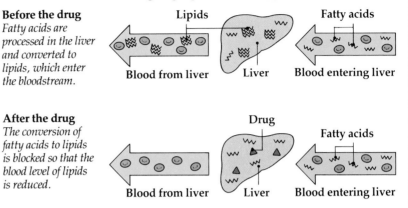

Before the drug
Fatty acids are processed in the liver and converted to lipids, which enter the bloodstream.

Lipids · Fatty acids · Blood from liver · Liver · Blood entering liver

After the drug
The conversion of fatty acids to lipids is blocked so that the blood level of lipids is reduced.

Drug · Fatty acids · Blood from liver · Liver · Blood entering liver

DRUGS THAT ACT ON THE BILE SALTS

These drugs reduce the reabsorption of bile salts into the bloodstream from the intestine. Because bile salts contain large amounts of cholesterol (a type of lipid), the effect of the drugs is to lower the level of lipids in the blood.

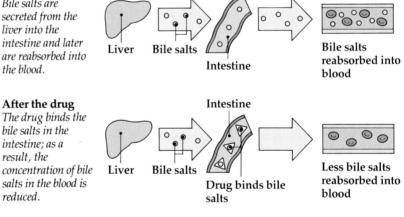

Before the drug
Bile salts are secreted from the liver into the intestine and later are reabsorbed into the blood.

Liver · Bile salts · Intestine · Bile salts reabsorbed into blood

After the drug
The drug binds the bile salts in the intestine; as a result, the concentration of bile salts in the blood is reduced.

Liver · Bile salts · Intestine · Drug binds bile salts · Less bile salts reabsorbed into blood

Would an overdose be dangerous?

An extra dose is unlikely to cause problems, but a large overdose may cause gastrointestinal disturbances; seek medical advice.

How long will I have to take the drugs?

Lipid-lowering drugs don't cure the underlying condition that causes hyperlipidemia, so you may have to take the drugs indefinitely.

COMMONLY PRESCRIBED LIPID-LOWERING DRUGS

Drugs that act on the liver

Clofibrate	Niacin
Gemfibrozil	Probucol
Lovastatin	

Drugs that act on the bile salts
Cholestyramine
Colestipol
Neomycin

DRUGS THAT AFFECT BLOOD CLOTTING

If you suffer from a disease of the blood vessels in which there is a tendency for blood clots to form, or if clots have already formed, your doctor may prescribe a drug that will prevent or disperse the clots. Diseases in which this tendency occurs include atherosclerosis (page 14) – whether it affects the arteries supplying the heart, the brain, or other parts of the body – and deep vein thrombosis (page 125).

Generally, clots form only at the site of an injury to a blood vessel. However, in atherosclerosis and deep vein thrombosis, abnormal clotting may occur and block a blood vessel, leading to a stroke, heart attack, or other circulatory problem such as gangrene of an extremity.

Types of drugs that affect blood clotting

Three types of drugs that affect blood clotting are used by doctors in the treatment of cardiovascular disease – antiplatelets, anticoagulants, and thrombolytics.

Antiplatelets

When there is an area of atheroma in a blood vessel, especially one of the fast-flowing blood vessels, platelets (small cells in the blood) tend to form sticky clumps around the atheroma. These clumps may develop into a blood clot. Antiplatelet drugs reduce the stickiness of the platelets, making them less likely to clump together and clot.

Antiplatelet drugs may be prescribed by your doctor after a heart valve replacement operation, or if you suffer from coronary heart disease (page 74) or from transient ischemic attacks (page 121). The most common antiplatelet regimen consists of low doses of aspirin.

Generally, antiplatelet drugs are not prescribed for children. Your doctor will prescribe them with caution if you suffer from a stomach ulcer or bleeding disorder, if you have impaired kidney or liver function, or if you are pregnant or breastfeeding. The use of antiplatelet drugs can reduce the severity and frequency of angina and help reduce the frequency of transient ischemic attacks. Some people taking antiplatelet medication experience nausea, vomiting, or indigestion.

Antiplatelet drugs are taken as tablets or capsules. In some cases, aspirin is administered as a rectal suppository. The frequency of the dose depends on your condition and the drug you are taking. Since antiplatelet drugs do not cure the underlying problem, they often need to be taken indefinitely.

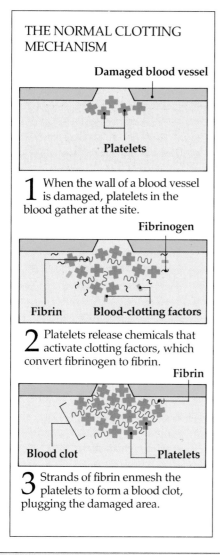

THE NORMAL CLOTTING MECHANISM

Damaged blood vessel

Platelets

1 When the wall of a blood vessel is damaged, platelets in the blood gather at the site.

Fibrinogen

Fibrin   **Blood-clotting factors**

2 Platelets release chemicals that activate clotting factors, which convert fibrinogen to fibrin.

Fibrin

Blood clot   **Platelets**

3 Strands of fibrin enmesh the platelets to form a blood clot, plugging the damaged area.

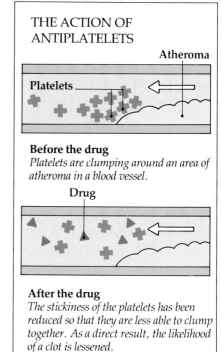

THE ACTION OF ANTIPLATELETS

Atheroma

Platelets

Before the drug
Platelets are clumping around an area of atheroma in a blood vessel.

Drug

After the drug
The stickiness of the platelets has been reduced so that they are less able to clump together. As a direct result, the likelihood of a clot is lessened.

Generally, missing a dose of the drug does not cause any problems; your doctor will tell you what to do if this happens. Some antiplatelet drugs are more potent than others, but any overdose should be treated as an emergency; get medical attention immediately.

Anticoagulants

If your blood has a tendency to form clots easily, or if you have just undergone surgery or been involved in an accident, your doctor may prescribe anticoagulant drugs to stabilize any existing clots and to try to prevent others from forming.

Anticoagulants interact with many other kinds of drugs, including aspirin, laxatives, and oral contraceptives. Always check with your doctor before taking any other medication if you are taking anticoagulants. Your doctor will prescribe anticoagulants with caution if you are pregnant or if you have impaired kidney or liver function.

Research studies on tens of thousands of patients have shown that anticoagulants do save lives, but their beneficial effects are rarely as noticeable as their side effects. You may find that you experience extra bruising, or occasional bleeding from the nose, gums, or urinary tract. You may also have digestive disturbances such as nausea.

Generally, you will take the drug orally as capsules or tablets, but occasionally an anticoagulant is injected intravenously in an emergency or before or after surgery. With many anticoagulants (particularly if you are taking warfarin), it is best to avoid alcohol, since it can increase the drug's effect beyond the desirable limit. Anticoagulants are usually prescribed for at least 6 months. In some cases, especially in people

THE ACTION OF ANTICOAGULANTS

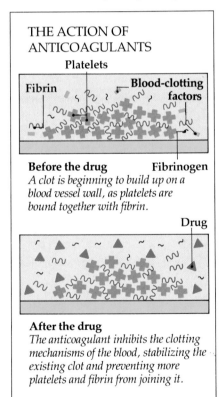

Platelets

Fibrin

Blood-clotting factors

Before the drug   **Fibrinogen**
A clot is beginning to build up on a blood vessel wall, as platelets are bound together with fibrin.

Drug

After the drug
The anticoagulant inhibits the clotting mechanisms of the blood, stabilizing the existing clot and preventing more platelets and fibrin from joining it.

who have an artificial heart valve, they may need to be taken indefinitely. During your treatment you will be given regular blood tests to ensure that the best dose for your condition is being prescribed; the dosage may be altered periodically.

If you miss a dose, it is unlikely to cause a problem; your doctor will tell

you exactly what to do. An overdose of anticoagulants is always a potential emergency, and medical help must be sought immediately.

Thrombolytics

When a blood clot forms in a blood vessel, it is bound together by strands of fibrin and normally cannot be broken down easily or rapidly. Thrombolytic drugs increase the blood level of plasmin, a substance that quickly breaks down the fibrin strands, so these drugs can be used to dissolve clots that have already formed. If you have had a heart attack (page 82), your doctor may inject a thrombolytic drug within a few hours of the attack to limit the damage to the heart and, ideally, to reopen a blocked coronary artery. Greatly enhanced survival rates are derived from these drugs only when they are given within 4 hours of the onset of the heart attack.

Women in the early months of pregnancy are given thrombolytic drugs only in a life-threatening situation because the drugs can cause the placenta of the developing baby to detach. Generally, the drugs are not prescribed for women who are at any stage of pregnancy or who are breast-feeding.

Thrombolytic drugs act very quickly and may dissolve an existing clot immediately. One side effect is an increased susceptibility to bruising and bleeding from even minor accidents. Streptokinase has been known to cause allergic reactions in some people. These reactions are treated with antihistamines and corticosteroid injections.

Thrombolytic drugs are usually administered in the hospital to clear specific clots; they may be given by intravenous infusion or may be injected directly into the affected blood vessel. Missed doses and overdoses are extremely unlikely because the treatment is so closely monitored. Thrombolytics are not used for long-term therapy.

THE ACTION OF THROMBOLYTICS

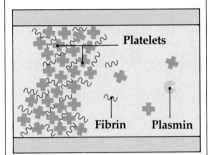

Platelets

Fibrin   **Plasmin**

Before the drug
A clot, formed of platelets meshed together by fibrin strands, is blocking a blood vessel. As a result, the flow of blood is interrupted.

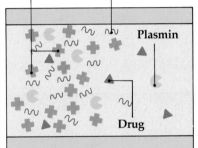

Platelets   **Fibrin**

Plasmin

Drug

After the drug
The drug increases the levels of plasmin in the blood. Plasmin quickly breaks down the fibrin strands and allows the blood clot to break up and disperse.

COMMONLY PRESCRIBED DRUGS THAT AFFECT BLOOD CLOTTING

Antiplatelets	**Anticoagulants**
Aspirin	Anisindione
Dipyridamole	Dicumarol
	Heparin
	Warfarin

Thrombolytics
Streptokinase
Tissue plasminogen activator (TPA)
Urokinase

DRUG INDEX

How to use the index

All entries in this index are generic names (recognized medical names) of drugs. All entries will cross-refer you either to one of the DRUG GROUPS on pages 128 to 137 or, in the case of a drug not belonging to any of these drug groups, to the TABLE on page 127. Brand names of drugs are not included in this index. If you have been prescribed a brand-name product, you can generally determine the generic name of its active ingredient or ingredients by reading the package insert.

A

acebutolol a beta blocker
adenosine an antiarrhythmic drug
alseroxylon a sympatholytic
amiloride a potassium-sparing diuretic
amiodarone an antiarrhythmic drug
amrinone a drug for heart failure
amyl nitrite a nitrate drug used to treat angina
anisindione an anticoagulant
anistreplase an investigational thrombolytic
aspirin a painkiller that is also effective as an antiplatelet drug
atenolol a beta blocker
atropine an antiarrhythmic drug

B

bendroflumethiazide a thiazide diuretic
benzthiazide a thiazide diuretic
bevantolol an investigational beta blocker
bezafibrate an investigational lipid-lowering drug
bretylium an antiarrhythmic drug
bumetanide a loop diuretic

C

captopril an ACE inhibitor used to treat hypertension and heart failure
carteolol a beta blocker
chlorothiazide a thiazide diuretic
chlorthalidone a thiazide diuretic
cholestyramine a lipid-lowering drug that acts on the bile salts
ciprofibrate an investigational lipid-lowering drug
clofibrate a lipid-lowering drug that acts on the liver
clonidine a sympatholytic
colestipol a lipid-lowering drug that acts on the bile salts
cyclandelate a drug for peripheral vascular disease
cyclothiazide a thiazide diuretic

D

deserpidine a sympatholytic
deslanoside a cardiac glycoside
diazoxide an antihypertensive drug for emergencies
dicumarol an anticoagulant
digitalis the active ingredient in cardiac glycosides

digitoxin a cardiac glycoside
digoxin a cardiac glycoside
diltiazem a calcium channel blocker
dipyridamole an antiplatelet drug
disopyramide an antiarrhythmic drug
dobutamine a drug used to treat heart failure
dopamine a drug for heart failure

E

edrophonium an antiarrhythmic drug
enalapril an ACE inhibitor
encainide an antiarrhythmic drug
epoprostenol an investigational antiplatelet and antiangina drug
erythrityl tetranitrate a nitrate
esmolol a beta blocker
ethacrynate sodium a loop diuretic
ethacrynic acid a loop diuretic
ethaverine a drug used for peripheral vascular disease

F

fenofibrate an investigational lipid-lowering drug
flecainide an antiarrhythmic drug

flumethiazide a thiazide diuretic
furosemide a loop diuretic

G

gemfibrozil a lipid-lowering drug that acts on the liver
guanabenz a sympatholytic
guanadrel a sympatholytic
guanethidine a sympatholytic
guanfacine a sympatholytic

H

heparin an anticoagulant
hydralazine an antihypertensive drug
hydrochlorothiazide a thiazide diuretic
hydroflumethiazide a thiazide diuretic

I

indapamide a thiazide diuretic
isoproterenol an antiarrhythmic drug
isosorbide dinitrate a nitrate
isoxsuprine a drug for peripheral vascular disease

K

ketanserin an investigational antihypertensive drug

L

labetalol a beta blocker
lidocaine a local anesthetic also used as an antiarrhythmic drug
lisinopril an ACE inhibitor
lovastatin a lipid-lowering drug that acts on the liver

M

mecamylamine a sympatholytic
methyclothiazide a thiazide diuretic
methyldopa a sympatholytic

metolazone a thiazide diuretic
metoprolol a beta blocker
metyrosine a sympatholytic
mexiletine an antiarrhythmic drug
milrinone a drug for heart failure
minoxidil an antihypertensive drug
moricizine an investigational anti-arrhythmic drug

N

nadolol a beta blocker
neomycin an antibiotic also used as a lipid-lowering drug, which acts on the bile salts
niacin a vitamin used as a lipid-lowering drug, which acts on the liver
nicardipine a calcium channel blocker
nifedipine a calcium channel blocker
nimodipine a calcium channel blocker
nitroglycerin a nitrate
nitroprusside see sodium nitroprusside
nylidrin a drug for peripheral vascular disease

P

penbutolol a beta blocker
pentaerythritol tetranitrate a nitrate
pentoxifylline a drug for peripheral vascular disease
phenoxybenzamine a sympatholytic
phentolamine a sympatholytic
phenytoin an anticonvulsant drug that has also been used as an anti-arrhythmic drug
pindolol a beta blocker
polythiazide a thiazide diuretic
prazosin a sympatholytic
probucol a lipid-lowering drug that acts on the liver
procainamide an antiarrhythmic drug
propafenone an investigational anti-arrhythmic drug
propranolol a beta blocker

Q

quinethazone a thiazide diuretic
quinidine an antiarrhythmic drug

R

rauwolfia serpentina a sympatholytic
rescinnamine a sympatholytic
reserpine a sympatholytic

S

sodium nitroprusside an antihypertensive drug
sotalol an investigational beta blocker
spironolactone a potassium-sparing diuretic
streptokinase a thrombolytic drug
sulfinpyrazone a drug for gout also used as an antiplatelet drug

T

terazosin a sympatholytic
ticlopidine an investigational antiplatelet drug
timolol a beta blocker
tissue plasminogen activator a thrombolytic drug
tocainide an antiarrhythmic drug
TPA see tissue plasminogen activator
triamterene a potassium-sparing diuretic
trichlormethiazide a thiazide diuretic
trimazosin an investigational sympatholytic
trimethaphan a sympatholytic used to reduce blood pressure in emergencies

U

urokinase a thrombolytic drug

V

verapamil a calcium channel blocker

W

warfarin an anticoagulant

GLOSSARY OF TERMS

Terms in *italics* in this glossary refer to other terms in the glossary.

A

Adams-Stokes disease
Repeated loss of consciousness due to insufficient blood flow to the brain as a result of a very rapid or very slow heartbeat.

Aneurysm
Ballooning of an *artery* due to a weakened area in its wall.

Angina
An oppressive heaviness or pain in the chest, also sometimes felt in the neck and arms.

Angiography
A procedure that enables blood vessels to be seen on film after they have been injected with a dye that is opaque to X-rays.

Angioplasty
The reconstruction or widening of the channel of a blood vessel.

Aorta
The main *artery* of the body.

Aortic valve
The valve that guards the opening of the left *ventricle* into the *aorta*.

Arrhythmia, cardiac
A disturbance of the rhythm or rate of the heartbeat.

Arterial
Pertaining to the *arteries*.

Arteriography
Angiography of the *arteries*.

Arteriole
A blood vessel that branches off an *artery* to link it to a *capillary*.

Arteriosclerosis
Disorders that cause loss of elasticity of the *artery* walls.

Arteritis
Inflammation of an *artery* wall, causing narrowing or obstruction of the artery and a reduction or cessation in blood flow.

Artery
A blood vessel that carries blood away from the heart.

Ascites
An excess of fluid in the abdomen.

Asystole
A term meaning the absence of heartbeat.

Atheroma
Fatty deposits under the inner lining of an *artery* that are associated with *atherosclerosis*.

Atherosclerosis
A disease of the *arteries* in which fatty deposits cause loss of elasticity and narrowing, and disrupt the flow of blood.

Atrioventricular node
A group of cells in the heart muscle that acts as a relay station for electrical impulses passing from the *atria* into the *ventricles*.

Atrium
Either of the two upper chambers of the heart.

B

Bradycardia
An adult heart rate of less than 60 beats per minute.

Bruits
The sounds made in the heart, *arteries*, or *veins* when blood circulation becomes turbulent or flows at an abnormal speed.

Bundle-branch block
A type of *heart block* in which the impulse to contract is delayed in the right or left *ventricle*.

C

Capillary
The smallest of the blood vessels. A network of capillaries carries blood between the smallest *arteries*, or *arterioles*, and the smallest *veins*, or *venules*.

Cardiac arrest
A cessation of the heart's pumping action.

Cardiac catheterization
The insertion of a delicate tube into the heart via a blood vessel to take measurements and to inject a contrast medium for imaging purposes.

Cardiology
The study of the heart's function and its disorders.

Cardiomegaly
Enlargement of the heart.

Cardiomyopathy
Any disease of the heart muscle that causes a reduction in the force of contractions.

Cardiovascular
Related to the heart and blood vessels.

Cardioversion
Another word for *defibrillation*.

Carditis
Inflammation of the heart or its lining.

Cerebrovascular disease
A disease of the brain resulting from a diseased *artery*.

Chordae tendineae
Delicate cords in the *ventricles* of the heart that tether the *mitral* and *tricuspid valves*.

Circulation
The continuous flow of blood throughout the body.

Claudication
A cramplike pain in the leg brought on by walking and relieved by rest.

Congenital
Meaning "present at birth."

Coronary care unit
A ward for acutely ill patients who have had a *myocardial infarction*.

Coronary heart disease
Malfunction of or damage to the heart caused by narrowing or blockage in one or more of the coronary *arteries*, which supply blood to the heart.

Coronary thrombosis
Blockage of one of the coronary *arteries*, which supply blood to the heart, by a *thrombus* (clot). This causes a section of the heart muscle to be deprived of oxygen, which causes it to die.

Cor pulmonale
Enlargement and failure of the right side of the heart due to a chronic lung disease that has increased resistance to blood flow through the *pulmonary artery*.

Cyanosis
A bluish color to the skin that is caused by insufficient oxygen in the blood; it is most noticeable on the lips and tongue, and in the nail beds.

D

Defibrillation
The administration of a brief electric shock to the heart to reverse some types of cardiac *arrhythmia*.

Dextrocardia
A rare *congenital* condition in which the heart is located in the right-hand side of the chest.

Diastole
The resting period of the heart muscle between contractions.

Ductus arteriosus
The blood vessel that enables blood to bypass the lungs in the fetus.

Dyspnea
Difficult or labored breathing.

Dysrhythmia, cardiac
Another word for *arrhythmia*.

E

Echocardiography
The use of ultrasound to image the structure of the heart.

Ectopic heartbeat
A heartbeat that is out of sequence with the normal rhythm.

Edema
Excess fluid in the body.

Electrocardiography
Recording and study of the electrical activity of the heart.

Embolism
Interruption to the flow of blood in an *artery*.

Endarterectomy
The surgical removal of the lining of an *artery* narrowed by *atherosclerosis* to restore normal blood flow.

Endocarditis
Inflammation of the *endocardium*.

Endocardium
The inner lining of the heart.

Epinephrine
A hormone released by the adrenal gland in conditions of stress, exercise, or fright.

F

Fibrillation
Rapid contractions of individual muscle fibers in the heart that cause the heart to produce an irregular, rapid rhythm.

Flutter
A type of *arrhythmia* in which there are rapid and ineffective contractions of the *atria*.

H

Heart attack
A *myocardial infarction*.

Heart block
An interruption of the passage of impulses through the conducting system of the heart.

Heart failure
The inability of the heart to maintain its work load of pumping blood to the lungs and the rest of the body.

Hypertension
A condition associated with repeated measurements of elevated blood pressure.

Hypotension
Low blood pressure that is almost never associated with trouble unless *shock* is present.

I

Infarction
The death of an area of tissue, caused by *ischemia*.

Ischemia
Lack of blood supply to an organ or tissue.

M

Mitral valve
The heart valve that guards the opening between the left *atrium* and left *ventricle*.

Murmur
The sound of turbulent blood flow through the heart, heard through a stethoscope.

Myocardial infarction
Death of part of the heart muscle, caused by loss of its blood supply. A large infarction may cause severe chest pain and sometimes a fatal *arrhythmia*. *Coronary thrombosis* is a common cause of a myocardial infarction.

Myocarditis
Inflammation of the heart.

Myocardium
The heart muscle.

Myxoma
A benign, jellylike tumor. Very rarely, a myxoma may grow inside the heart, in which case it can lead to intermittent obstruction of the flow of blood.

O

Orthopnea
Breathing difficulty noted when lying flat.

P

Pacemaker
A device used to stimulate, or control the rate of, the heartbeat.

Palpitation
Awareness of the heartbeat.

Patent
Meaning open or unobstructed.

Pericarditis
Inflammation of the *pericardium*, often leading to chest pain and fever.

Pericardium
The membrane enclosing the heart and the roots of the major vessels that emerge from it.

Phlebitis
Inflammation of a *vein*.

Pressure points
Points on the body at which *arteries* lie near the surface and where pressure can be applied to control *arterial* bleeding.

Pulmonary
Pertaining to the lungs.

Pulmonary artery
The *artery* that carries blood out of the heart and to the lungs.

Pulmonary embolism
Obstruction of the *pulmonary artery* or one of its branches by an embolus.

Pulmonary valve
The heart valve that guards the opening of the right *ventricle* into the *pulmonary artery*.

Pulmonary vein
A *vein* that returns blood to the heart from the lungs.

Pulse
The rhythmic expansion and contraction of an *artery* as blood is pumped through it.

S

Sclerosis
Hardening of any body tissue, commonly used to refer to hardening of the blood vessels, as in *atherosclerosis*.

Shock
A dangerous reduction in blood flow that may occur in any situation in which blood vessels are abnormally widened, in which blood flow is obstructed, or in which the heart's pumping action is severely weakened.

Sinoatrial node
Specialized cells in the heart that emit electrical impulses.

Stenosis
Narrowing of a duct or a canal.

Stroke
Interruption in the blood supply to the brain, causing impaired sensation, movement, vision, or speech.

Syncope
The medical term for fainting.

Systole
The period of contraction of the heart muscle.

T

Tachycardia
An abnormally rapid heart rate of more than 100 beats per minute.

Tamponade
Compression of the heart.

Thrill
Vibration felt when the hand is placed on the chest wall over the heart when there is substantial turbulence of blood flow.

Thrombosis
The formation of a clot inside an intact blood vessel.

Transient ischemic attack
A brief interruption to the brain's blood supply that results in temporarily impaired sensation, movement, vision, or speech.

Tricuspid valve
The heart valve that guards the opening between the right *atrium* and right *ventricle*.

V

Vagus nerve
A nerve that transmits signals from the brain to the heart and to many other body organs.

Valvotomy or valvulotomy
An operation to open up a narrowed heart valve.

Vasculitis
Inflammation of the blood vessels.

Vasoconstriction
Narrowing (produced by nerve or hormonal stimulation) of one or many blood vessels.

Vasodilation
Widening of one or many blood vessels.

Vasovagal attack
Sudden slowing of the heartbeat brought on by pain, stress, shock, or fear, leading to temporary loss of consciousness.

Vein
A vessel that returns blood from various organs of the body to the heart.

Vena cava
Either of two very large veins – the superior vena cava and the inferior vena cava – into which all the blood drains before being delivered to the right *atrium*.

Venipuncture
The piercing of a *vein* with a needle to withdraw blood or inject fluid.

Venography
Angiography of the *veins*.

Ventricle
Either of the two lower, stronger, thicker-walled chambers of the heart.

Venule
Any of the small blood vessels that collect blood from the *capillaries* and join to form *veins*.

INDEX

Page numbers in *italics* refer to illustrations and captions. For listing, information, and indexing of specific drugs used for heart and circulatory disorders, see DRUG INDEX on pages 138–139.

Photograph sources:
Ace Photo Agency 47
The Image Bank **13** (top right); **16** (center left)
Mallinckrodt Institute of Radiology **58** (center); **72** (top)
National Medical Slide Bank, UK **68** (inset); **68** (bottom); **104** (top); **104** (center); **104** (bottom); **122** (bottom right); **123**; **124**
Pictor International **19**; **24** (bottom)
Barry Richards **13** (top left); **13** (center left); **13** (center right); **13** (bottom right); **79** (top); **79** (bottom right); **88** (bottom left); **89** (top right); **96** (top); **100** (center); **100** (bottom left); **100** (bottom right); **101** (top); **101** (center); **101** (bottom)
Royal Postgraduate Medical School, Hammersmith Hospital **54** (bottom left); **54** (bottom center); **93** (top right); **119** (center); **119** (bottom)
Saint Bartholomew's Hospital **117** (center right)
Science Photo Library **2** (top); **2** (bottom left); **2** (bottom right); **7**; **14**; **17** (top right); **33**; **37** (center); **40** (bottom center); **40** (bottom right); **41** (top right); **41** (center right); **53** (center); **54** (bottom right); **56** (center); **57**; **58** (top); **58** (bottom); **59** (top); **59** (center); **60**; **63** (center); **65**; **71** (center left); **75** (bottom left); **76** (bottom); **89** (bottom right); **90** (bottom left); **91** (bottom); **93** (top left); **96** (bottom); **97** (center left); **103** (top); **107** (right); **109**; **113** (top center); **113** (top right); **113** (center left); **113** (bottom); **114** (bottom right); **116**; **118**; **120**; **122** (bottom left)
Siemens **56** (top)
Dr P. Sweny **55** (center); **113** (center right)
Tony Stone Worldwide **9**; **12** (top right); **16** (bottom right)
Dr Robert Youngson **113** (top right)

Health campaign posters "Love Your Heart" (1984) and "Eat smart" (1986) on page 12 reproduced with permission from the American Heart Association.

Commissioned photography:
Stephen Oliver
Susanna Price
Barry Richards
Clive Streeter

Illustrators:
Russell Barnet
Karen Cochrane
Graham Corbett
David Fathers
Tony Graham
Andrew Green

Coral Mula
Lynda Payne
Howard Pemberton
Lydia Umney
John Woodcock

Airbrushing:
Roy Flooks
Trevor Hill
Janos Marffy
Roger Stewart

Charts:
Technical Art Services